Visit our website

to find out about other books from (Baillière Tindall)
and our sister companies in Harcourt Health Sciences

Register free at
www.harcourt-international.com

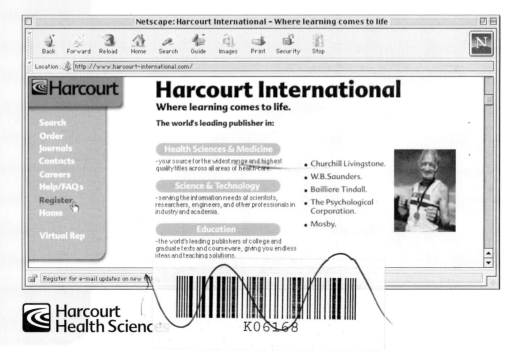

Holistic Stoma Care

Patricia K Black MSc, SRN, RCNT
Clinical Specialist, Stoma Care, Hillingdon Health Authority, Hillingdon, UK

Foreword by

John E L Sales MA Mchir FRCS

Baillière Tindall
PUBLISHED IN ASSOCIATION WITH THE RCN

N Royal College
of Nursing

EDINBURGH LONDON NEW YORK PHILADELPHIA ST LOUIS SYDNEY TORONTO 2000

BAILLIÈRE TINDALL
An imprint of Harcourt Publishers Limited

© Harcourt Publishers Limited 2000

❀ is a registered trademark of Harcourt Publishers Limited

The right of Patricia K Black to be identified as author of this work has been asserted by her in accordance with the Copyright, Designs and Patents Act 1988

First published 2000

ISBN 07020 2304 3

British Library Cataloguing in Publication Data
A catalogue record for this book is available from the British Library

Library of Congress Cataloging in Publication Data
A catalog record for this book is available from the Library of Congress

Note
Medical knowledge is constantly changing. As new information becomes available, changes in treatment, procedures, equipment and the use of drugs become necessary. The author and the publishers have taken care to ensure that the information given in this text is accurate and up to date. However, readers are strongly advised to confirm that the information, especially with regard to drug usage, complies with the latest legislation and standards of practice.

The publisher's policy is to use paper manufactured from sustainable forests

Printed in China

Contents

Foreword

When I was appointed to Hillingdon Hospital in 1973 there was no stoma therapist on the staff. In my first clinic I found a lady who had had a stoma for 10 years and who had never seen or worn a bag!

Prior to my appointment to Hillingdon I was a senior registrar to Ian Todd at St Bartholomew's Hospital. In 1969 he had set up a monthly clinic with his ward sister, Barbara Saunders, to look after the special needs of stoma patients. In 1971 she was appointed as the first stoma care nurse in the UK. She initiated the first training courses for stoma therapists, so I was fortunately able to appoint a stoma therapist within 2 years of my arrival at Hillingdon Hospital.

Since those early days, the stoma therapist has become a highly skilled member of the colo-proctology team, providing both hospital and domiciliary care to stoma patients. The devel-opment of pouch surgery has given the stoma therapist another important role. Most patients with pouches take up to 12 months to acculturate after the construction of the pouch, and during this period the regular support of the stoma therapist is vital.

It has been a great pleasure to work with Pat Black over the past 15 years. My patients have benefited from her well-organised, highly skilled and sympathetic care. In addition to her hospital work, she has been in demand worldwide as a lecturer and has also published many papers on stoma care.

This book is an excellent distillation of her knowledge and wide experience of stoma care. I am sure it will be of benefit to coloproctologists and nursing staff.

John E. L. Sales, MA, Mchir, FRCS, 2000

Preface

Today, there is no doubt that patients who have to undergo stoma surgery are able to adapt to their new body image and way of life provided that there is professional and voluntary input, from the preoperative stage through to rehabilitation and return to the community to lead a normal and productive life. The shock of realisation for a patient who arrives home with only limited (if any) professional help and training is incalculable. For some patients, the only ongoing point of contact after return home is a general practitioner who signs the repeat prescription, rarely sees the patient, and would find it difficult to find the time to deal with any physical and psychological problems experienced by the patient.

Nursing has moved away from the role of mechanistic, task-orientated care – in this instance caring for the stoma – and now considers the patient as a whole. There are many more areas to be taken into account apart from the obvious physical changes and any problems they may bring. Cultural background plays an important part in patient's lives, including their beliefs (whether personal or religious), perceptions, behaviours, concepts and their attitudes to disease, illness and pain. Socioeconomic factors also have a role to play in the patient's well-being, and doctors and nurses are sometimes surprised to discover that some patients do not have indoor toilets, hot water or washing facilities, or that they live with 20 other families and share one toilet, or even have to walk to a toilet facility in a concrete block with only cold water and no electric light. How can a patient with a newly formed stoma be expected to cope in situations such as these if the nurse has not enquired what the patient's expectations are for discharge planning and does not understand the culture from which the patient comes? Patients from ethnic minorities are never homogeneous and generalisations in their care should not be made. There may be rules that govern how a culture thinks and behaves, but how people react under the stress of disease and illness – and for some impending death – can lead to misunderstandings for nursing and medical staff and generate feelings of lack of care for patients and their families.

The first section of this book endeavours to help the practitioner to think in a wider-ranging way and to consider the patient's culture, socioeconomic situation, beliefs, religion and any practices that relate to ill health. Patients diagnosed with colorectal cancer or inflammatory bowel disease may link their illness to a misfortune that has befallen them such as personal problems, personal body abuse (i.e. smoking, alcohol or drugs), accidents or eating the 'wrong' food. Patients from some societies and ethnic minorities may blame their illness on supernatural forces, crop failures or witchcraft, which for the Western doctor or nurse, working in an ethnocentric, biomedical situation, is difficult to understand. Without an understanding of the culture in which patients have grown up, the practitioner will have difficulty in understanding their reaction to disease and illness, particularly in stoma surgery, which can leave both patient and practitioner frustrated with the care-giving and care-receiving process.

Research in nursing is increasingly incorporated into the daily work of many clinical nurses. The importance of using research and evidence based care to direct the care of the patient has never been so great as it is in today's litigious health service. The last section of the book looks at ethics and evidence based care in stoma care. Evidence based care and research help both the promotion of good nursing care and the understanding of failures in practice, with the aim of rectifying the situation. Patients such as stoma patients are vulnerable and are in a relationship with the doctor and nurse in which there is an inherent imbalance of power – the patient trusts the nurse to give the best possible care based on up-to-date knowledge and research. Nurses have an obligation to keep up with the literature in their field, to read it critically, and to make balanced judgements about the quality and relevance of the work in relation to their practice.

Today, health care research is moving away from the biomedical approach and quantitative research towards qualitative research. Qualitative research seeks to find a deeper meaning and to study things in their natural surroundings by attempting to make sense of or interpret phenomena, patterns or characteristics that make the phenomena what they are. Qualitative research includes documenting and fully describing experiences, rituals, life situations and other aspects that are of importance to the patient and allow the practitioner entrance to the patient's world. The goal, therefore, of qualitative research is to interpret fully the totality of what is being studied from the patient's viewpoint. Qualitative research uses a holistic perspective which preserves the complexities of human nature. In stoma care, qualitative research comes into its own, being used to examine uncharted territory where variables of greatest concern are often poorly understood, ill defined and out of the nurse's control. Using the iterative approach allows nurses to be sensitive to the richness and variability of their subject matter.

So where will stoma care be going in the new millennium? Concern that many experienced and expert practitioners are leaving practice based posts to advance their careers and earnings has led the government to announce that by April 2000 there will be the first appointments of nurse consultants. The establishment of nursing consultant posts is intended to provide better outcomes for patients by improving services and quality, strengthening leadership, and providing a new career opportunity for experienced and expert nurses. There is no reason why these posts cannot be established in a speciality. So, will there be nurse consultants in stoma care in 2000? In taking the nurse consultant post further forward, there may eventually be regional nurses in stoma care using their expertise and experience across several trusts, budgeting and making decisions on appliance buying and patient care. Within the primary and secondary care areas there might be colorectal facilitators who would work at the clinical level caring for patients and their families. Nurse consultants in stoma care are perhaps not yet a reality, but then, in 1970 neither were specialist nurses in stoma care.

PKB, 2000

Acknowledgements

In taking on a project such as this, one needs constant encouragement and support, especially when it seems that everything is conspiring against completion. There are, needless to say, many people who have shown an interest in the project over the last 2 years and who have helped in their various ways, including many friends in the ostomy industry, past and present.

But there are certain people who give constant help and support, who continually check that all is going to plan, and my grateful thanks go to:

Keith Filmer, Val and John Howberry Gale, Barbara Stuchfield, John Sales, Peter Mitchenere, Jane Walton, Yvonne and Ray South, Samira Mumani and George Quayson.

I am especially grateful to Claire Davidson for all her sterling work, under great difficulty, in the transcribing of the early sections, and to both Claire and Christine Hyde for putting up with my computer illiteracy and ill-timed telephone calls!

PKB, 2000

The construction of illness and its interpretation

1

Body image

The social taboos that surround body matter elimination are legion, so that when a stoma (from classical Greek *stoma*, meaning 'mouth', medical 'artificial opening') is raised as a surgical procedure, in order to eliminate faeces or urine onto the outside abdominal wall, the individual's body image changes forever. Body image, the mental picture of their physical being that individuals retain, develops from birth onwards and continues throughout life, and is related to different factors affecting its formation and dynamics. A crisis such as the creation of a stoma leads to an alteration of body image and an awareness of the meaning of the change in appearance and function of an individual (Black 1992). The individual's behaviour is examined in several domains: physical, cognitive, emotional, cultural, sexual and economic. Feelings of violation of the body boundaries, degradation, mutilation and restriction occur. The intensity of emotional reactions to body changes are related less to the severity of the disability than to the assigned importance of the structure, and this appraisal depends, among other factors, on the individual's immediate social situation and past experiences. It follows that the importance assigned to function will also be a determinant in the severity of the emotional reaction.

Many factors affect the patient's ability to adapt to an alteration in body image, and these are relevant to both the patient and the patient's family. These factors include, but are not limited to, the disease process, diagnosis, treatment and medical and nursing care within the hospital and on return to the community. Most people feel that bodily elimination is a private function, best managed in one's own home. This can be related to the common notion that dirt is harmful both to the individual and others. Douglas (1966) stated that: 'Dirt is essentially disorder. Dirt offends against order. Eliminating it is not a negative movement but a positive effort to organise the environment.'

By reordering our environment we make it conform to an idea. An individual with a stoma sees him- or herself as a person who has transgressed certain social expectations and failed in certain personal responsibilities. Bodily excretion can be used as the schema for suggesting that individuals are 'in' or 'out' of control of themselves or are being controlled by others. Orifices of the body, located as they are at the margins between the self and the external world, serve as particularly apt symbols for the boundaries of the community. Douglas (1966) reports that sometimes bodily orifices seem to represent points of entry or exit to social units and that bodily perfection can symbolise an ideal purity. Douglas proposes that no one knows how long ideas of purity and impurity have been established in any non-literate culture, but to its members they must seem timeless and unchanging. However, there is every reason to believe that such ideas are in fact sensitive to change. Provisional recognition of anomaly leads to anxiety and from there to suppression or avoidance.

Excretion and excretory behaviour are rigidly controlled in each culture and in each society, and in Western societies there are strong prohibitions on the uncontrolled passage of urine and faeces. It is often considered that personality too is altered through a link with excreta, as in such statements as 'the mean and parsimonious man is anally retentive'. The structure and functions of the human body provide a locus onto which meanings can be placed. A specific type of behaviour can have many meanings, and in order to disambiguate meaning, a culturally distinctive interpretative theory is needed to transform natural behaviour into the behaviour of the social being. Within both Egyptian cosmology, and Western thought, excrement can represent the potential

for fertilisation and, within the latter, the understanding of the nitrogen cycle. Prohibitions concerned with excrement are numerous, and it has been associated with madness, danger and witchcraft. To excrete through a different body exit requires a specific schema, which the individual and his society must understand if the individual is not to become a marginal member of that society. The Western world enforces rigid laws in association with the civilised disposal of human waste by means of the private act of excretion, and the raising of a stoma can risk placing the individual in a liminal position, as dangerous to society, as mentioned above.

Loudon (1977) considers that babies soon find out that they can obtain the approval of mother and father by producing faeces at the right time and in the right place, or disapproval if the time and the place are wrong, while refusing to produce faeces at all can inflict pain, not only on themselves but also on those closest to them, and thus reciprocity is gradually learned. Achieving continence is regarded as one of the major milestones of childhood. The need to ask for permission to use a bedpan or to get up to use the toilet sometimes experienced by the ill person admitted to hospital can be interpreted as a partial return of the sick person to the early stage of infancy, to being controlled and liable to humiliation, especially if the bedpan is slow in coming and the sheets become dirtied by incontinence. The consideration that one function of the nurse is as a symbolic mother is to use culturally understood meanings of need, both professional and lay, and is there to disambiguate the patient's tentative signal. As human beings we draw boundaries between ourselves and the outside world – when these boundaries break down we find it profoundly disturbing, and when something in the system we have conceived breaks down it violates something intrinsic to our sense of ourselves.

Most people deal with this disturbance by denying what is happening. Littlewood (1985) suggests that in Western culture, if one can define oneself as sick when acts of excretion occur in the wrong place, they can be forgiven or managed in such a way as to ensure that the transgressor is not socially ostracised. If one is not able to declare oneself sick, either because one cannot, or because one does not wish to do so, incontinence can reduce one to a childlike state.

The process through which people come to construct or reorder meaning in their sickness experiences has been analysed by several classic medical anthropologists. One well-known dominant perspective is that of explanatory models of illness (Good 1977, Kleinman 1980). Explanatory models (EMs) help people to create order and meaning in sickness situations and provide indications for purposive action. Kleinman considered that explanatory models are not likely to be homogenous, but rather that they are related to individuals and that they change over time in relation to people's sickness experiences. They can make useful models for trying to control and predict what may happen in relation to the experience of sickness in various health care settings.

The individual who loses control over bodily elimination is presented with sensory phenomena (sounds, odour) which were previously within his or her control (Klopp 1990). In addition to the person's own perception of these phenomena (actual or potential), the social perception of the phenomena becomes an issue, because of their very nature. We learn to control elimination at an early age, in private, so that exteriorising the bodily structures we use for elimination and loss of control over the accompanying sensory phenomena inevitably results in a changed body image.

Littlewood (1991) has published the experience of incontinence of one particular patient:

but incontinence is not merely embarrassing, it is shaming and ignominious. I can still recall with painful clarity just after my difficulties walking along the road I would suddenly feel the urgent desire to empty my bowels. I would stop for a moment to assess how far I was from home. Sweat would break out as I was desperately trying to decide what course of action to take. Would it be better to hurry and reach safety as quickly as possible, bearing in mind that hurrying would further excite my gut, or should I slow down, which would be just as disturbing to my insides but prolong the time to get to the toilet? Even if I couldn't get to the lavatory could I at least get through my own front door before the noises, stains, and smells broadcast my predicament to the outside world?

Sometimes I could not and my feeling of degradation was complete. I would stand for ages in the shower where the tears streaming down my face would not show.

Many patients with colitis, before their surgical operation, express similar feelings and experience a sense of degradation or humiliation when out and about, perhaps unable to find a toilet quickly and having to take with them many changes of underwear in case there should be a disaster. Some patients who have failed to come to terms with a change in body image after a stoma also have a similar experience. Some feel unsafe to go out, worried that the appliance will be unreliable, that it will leak, that they will need to take extra clothing, and that they still need to find every toilet within a very small radius of their home area. Unfortunately there are still patients who refuse to go out after their stoma surgery, becoming reclusive, although nowadays, with the number of stoma care nurses and the input of excellent counselling both pre- and postoperatively, they are fewer in number.

Within society, the human body can serve as a symbol for the social body: the body in health offers a model of wholeness, the body in sickness offers a model of social disharmony, conflict and disintegration. As discussed above, the change in body image brought about by stoma surgery is analogous with a rite of passage, one which is not purifactory but prophylactic.

The individual's status within society is not being restored but redefined, and while being redefined passes through a transitional state which is deemed by society to be dangerous. After stoma surgery has been undergone, anxiety, or even terror, are expressed in relation to pollution beliefs. Although pollution beliefs are a cultural phenomenon, fear is exhibited by individuals in understanding how they will be able to modify their behaviour and hide their stigma on return to the culture and society in which they live (Goffman 1963).

In seeking to evaluate the possible benefits to patients of specialised care such as that provided by the stoma care nurse specialist, it is important to identify the specific areas most likely to affect patient outcome. After stoma surgery, the most important area is certainly the adaptation of patients to their change of body image, both internally and externally. In seeking to derive a framework it is necessary to consider the implications of stoma surgery (Murray 1972).

The sources of stress to patients admitted to hospital, especially those undergoing surgery, have been described by many researchers, among them Cohen & Lazarus (1982). For the patient undergoing stoma surgery additional sources of stress arise: threats to body integrity, permanent physical damage, loss of autonomy and control and a diagnosis of cancer are some of the uncertainties that stoma patients and their carers fear. Kelly (1985) graphically recalls his feelings:

the protruding stoma and its attachments looked horrible, moreover I now realised how uncontrollable it was and what being permanently incontinent implied. What really alarmed me were the physiological consequences, especially the incontinence and the smell. These I believed would become the defining characteristics of my social identity and everything about me, my relationships, the way others viewed me would be conditioned by these.

The suggestion by Van Gennep (1909) discussed above, that rites of transition, treating marginal or ill-defined states as dangerous, compare to the sociological approach to pollution, but also edges and boundaries such as body boundaries which are used in the order of social experience and are treated as dangerous or polluting. They are prophylactic only and not purifactory, and do not redefine and restore a lost former status or purify from the effects of contamination but define entrance to a new status.

When an individual presents him- or herself to others, the group will seek to acquire information about that individual or to redefine information they already possess. Such information helps the group to define a situation, and enables both the individual and the group to know in advance what to expect of each other. Many sources of information are available to the group, including sign vehicles, body language and the individual's general conduct and appearance. The individual communicates with the group by means of the visual evidence he or she presents – clothes, stance, reactions – but individuals with stomas will automatically feel that they do not fit the group stereotype, since their body boundaries have been transgressed. They will also be aware that there are phenomena which may occur over which they can have no control.

Chesterfield defined 'dirt' as matter out of place, and this implies that there is a set of ordered relations and a contravention of that order. The underlying feeling is that a system of cultural values that is habitually expressed in a certain arrangement has been violated. Often individuals who have undergone stoma surgery consider themselves stigmatised, a term used by the Greeks to refer to bodily signs indicating something unusual and bad about the moral status of the person so marked. Modern medicine uses the term to refer to the bodily signs of a physical disorder, but it is more generally applied to the disgrace rather than to the bodily evidence of it. As noted earlier, Douglas (1966) suggested that the orifices of the body, being located at the margin between the self and the external world, serve as apt symbols of the community. Excretion is considered, therefore, to be ambiguous, being both part and not part of the individual, passing from the individual's internal to external self via margins of the physical body. The strong prohibitions on the uncontrolled passage of urine and faeces in Western societies, suggests Littlewood (1991), may be due to the value placed on a post-Cartesian self compared with the socially contextual and reverential notion of the self in non-literate societies.

Although profound distortions in body image are rare, there are many anxieties about the body and its image in relationship to its orifices, boundaries and bodily fluids. Stigmatisation by exteriorising excretory organs, especially later in life, may lead an individual to have problems with the reidentification of self, or to the development of a disapproval of self. This may be expressed in distortion of the total self, giving rise to confusion and negative changes in an individual's self-perceptions. People whose previous self-esteem was unrealistically high, or those who take great pride in their appearance and care very much how others perceive them will find it more difficult to accept changes in body image and presentation of self. A stoma which is disfiguring to the body will probably be more disfiguring to the mind. In addition, violation of the body's intactness can be perceived at a fantasy level as physical or sexual assault.

Kelly (1985) describes his fears of the possible effects on friends and work colleagues:

For the rest of the day I felt utterly wretched, sad and overwhelmed by a sense of loss and failure. I was not upset by the loss of my bowel per se but rather by the loss of its function. The sense of failure came from viewing my body as being wrecked by surgery. What really alarmed me were the physiological consequences, especially the incontinence and the smell. These I believed would become the defining characteristics of my social identity and everything about me, my relationships, and the way others viewed me would be conditioned by these.

The major consideration in terms of adaptation to the change in body image after stoma surgery would seem to be the length of time the grieving process takes. Parkes (1972) outlined the stages which appear to occur in all individuals with a change in body image:

1. *Realisation*: characterised by avoidance or denial of the loss followed by experiences of unreality or blunting
2. *Alarm*: characterised by anxiety, restlessness, fear and insecurity
3. *Searching*: characterised by acute episodic feelings of anxiety and panic and preoccupation with loss
4. *Grief*: characterised by feelings of internal loss and mutilation
5. *Resolution*: characterised by efforts to construct a new social identity.

When boundaries between self and cosmology break down it can be profoundly disturbing, and the individual then utilises the coping mechanisms described by Parkes.

In the immediate postoperative period people who have undergone stoma surgery will need help in caring for their changed condition. The nurse, represented by her uniform, is seen as being symbolically pure, and because of this symbolism is protected from pollution by dirt. Sharing dirt depends on knowledge and friendship – the more intimate one is the greater the sharing. To share or care for the pollution of others is a restatement of humility and love (Dunlop 1986). The nurse is expected to clean up bodily secretions, and this is seen as 'her' dirt as opposed to 'ward' dirt, dust, spills and so on. Nurses become identified with personal pollution and the individual's transgression of social codes. At this stage of body change and re-identification, the individual is in an ambiguous state and the nurse's presence is protective. Perception by the individual before stoma surgery is built into organised patterns for which the perceiver is responsible. As perceivers, elected stimuli falling on senses are schematically determined and this produces a schema for living. As time goes on these experiences accumulate and a system of labelling is used within the schema, but the individual who has undergone a body image change will have to modify the structure of assumptions to accommodate new experiences. The more consistent the past experiences of an individual, the more confidence he or she will have in rebuilding his or her schema.

A literature search about the experiences of patients with a stoma and their adaptation to their new lifestyle and to body image changes shows a number of common themes. As far back as 1956, Dyk & Sutherland were saying that an immense price is paid for the cure, and that this price incorporates not only physical discomfort, but also psychological and social trauma. Devlin et al (1971) looked at the effect of surgery after colorectal cancer and found how devastated the patients with a colostomy were and how life could be quite complicated. Padilla & Grant (1985) suggested that there is a relationship between the quality of life and self-esteem among individuals with stomas. The outcome of their study showed that the quality of life and self-esteem were indicative and that overall the ostomate population had positive perceptions. It was also suggested that individuals with stomas have poor psychosocial recovery outcomes that can include not returning to their previous occupation, reclusiveness and not wanting contact with friends or sometimes even family.

Wade (1990) points out that a patient facing stoma surgery also faces the prospect of a change in appearance and loss of control of elimination. From the mid-1970s onwards an increasing number of stoma care nurses have become specialists in their own right, and at the time of writing, at the end of the 1990s, there are considerable numbers of stoma care nurses in the UK. Wade suggests, however, that even with all this increased input of care, patients who have a stoma remain afraid of rejection by friends and family and of being ostracised by society. Rejection by sexual partners and breakdown of marriage may also occur.

2

Explanatory models and semantic networks

EXPLANATORY MODELS

Both patients and health care practitioners have preconceived ideas about patterns of illness and of how illness should be interpreted and treated. Kleinman (1981) describes five core points used to distinguish these notions about episodes of sickness and treatment. He calls these the core clinical functions of how systems of medical knowledge and practice enable people to:

- Culturally construct illness as a psychosocial experience
- Establish general criteria to guide the health-seeking process and to evaluate the treatment approach
- Manage particular illness episodes by communication, labelling and explaining
- Engage in healthy activities and therapeutic interventions, medicine, surgery, healing rituals and counselling
- Manage the therapeutic outcome and appropriate treatments for the condition.

These five care points or notions about sickness and illness have been described by Kleinman as explanatory models (EMs). The clinical process is one way for the individual to adapt to certain worrying circumstances, for example the formation of a stoma. The adaptation premise is reflected in Kleinman's choice of words such as 'guiding', 'managing', 'coping', 'explaining' and 'negotiating alliances' (Young 1982).

The cultural construction of an illness can often be a personal and social adaptive response.

Malfunctioning of the body and the psychological processes involved become disease, and the psychosocial disruption becomes illness. Illness will involve cognition, evaluation of the symptoms and possible breakdown of family and social interaction. Therefore illness is the shaping of disease into behaviour and experience and is created by personal, social and cultural reactions to the disease. The first stage of healing is a construction of illness from disease to form a coping function. Intentionally there are instances in which constructional reordering of cultural meaning may be all that the therapy consists of. By asserting the complementary nature of mind and body, healing and curing, Kleinman and his associates reject the crude Cartesianism of the biomedical model of sickness (Young 1982).

Explanatory models are not new to Western biomedicine. Practitioners of healing have existed for as long as professional functions have been specialised in human society and medical lore is integral to every existing human culture (Leslie 1976). Comparisons of the healer or medicine man within a culture have to be understood in a cultural context. Healers have often been called to the role by personal experience. They have acquired arcane knowledge, and are deemed to have great powers. Their principal social function is to diagnose and prescribe ritual actions to overcome illness or form a prognosis – they name and explain and form explanatory models. Since all belief systems are culture bound, little sense can be made of them out of context. They will also change as the society in which they exist changes and as newer beliefs displace, merge, or coexist with the society's older beliefs.

The lay explanatory model is put together in response to a particular episode of illness and is not the same as the individual's general beliefs about illness that his or her society may hold. By contrast, the physicians' explanatory model is based on scientific logic and deals with a single cause. Doctor and patient, each using his or her own explanatory model, must agree about the interpretation of each model, the individual's subjective view of the illness and the doctor's view of the disease process. Any problems must be resolved by negotiation so that the patient will comply with the prescribed treatment. (See also Fig. 2.1, below.)

Even today, in our modern industrial society, a large number of folk illnesses persist, many of them untouched by the medical model and still firmly rooted in traditional folklore. Conditions such as cancer, heart disease, and now especially AIDS, are sometimes linked in the public imagination with traditional beliefs about the moral nature of health, illness and suffering. These anxiety-provoking diseases have come to symbolise people's more general anxieties and fears, such as fear of the breakdown of an ordered society, of an invasion or of divine punishment or retribution. Susan Sontag (1978), in her book *Illness as metaphor*, describes how certain serious diseases – especially those whose origin was not understood and whose treatment was not very successful – historically became metaphors for all that was unnatural in society and socially or morally wrong. Diseases such as tuberculosis, syphilis and cancer were used as contemporary metaphors of evil. In the 20th century cancer in particular has been described in the media and in literature as if it were a type of unrestrained Celtic evil force unique to the modern world, a disease in which cells behave completely without inhibition and which can destroy the natural order of the body and of society. Metaphors of ill health, especially when they are attached to serious conditions such as colorectal cancer and inflammatory bowel disease, can carry with them a range of associations which can affect how sufferers perceive their condition and how people behave towards them. Bowel movement, for example, is associated with an opening up, allowing entry into the body, the opposite of closing. Assorted words used here are 'empty', 'loosen up', 'unblock', and these suggest that a change has taken place in the internal space of the gut. Having one's bowels emptied is a physical reality associated with the control of internal space and purity – the person is made clean because the bowels are empty. This is often seen when bowel prep is given prior to bowel surgery so that the doctor may have unimpeded access to the organ. It is often said that people 'locate' themselves in their bowels

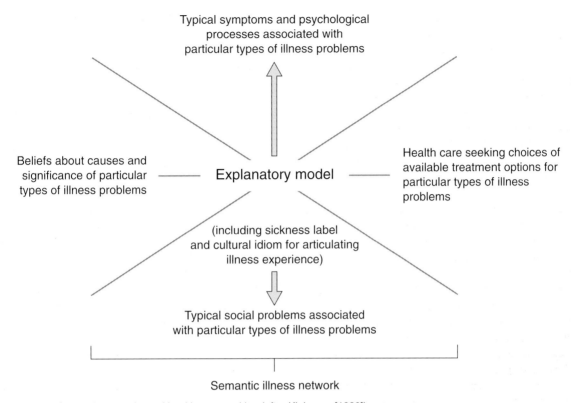

Figure 2.1   Semantic networks and health care seeking (after Kleinman [1980])

and it is considered that the removal of the contents of the bowel may be parallel to removal of self, becoming void, nothing. Foucault (1976) suggested that the person becomes not only clean or in control, but also someone who is no one, who is seen as a symbolic part of the body of the ward, which is in turn a piece of the body of the hospital which is sliced into bits for medical gaze. The basic very personal and private functioning of the individual's bowels in the public domain is also a defining boundary. Young (1981) has suggested that these metaphors of illness emerge at times when understanding is experiential and empirical.

In Western society, if an organ is not functioning properly, or is diseased, it is often viewed as 'not self'. The patient will say 'I'm all right, nurse, but my bowels aren't'. The diseased part is taken out of the description of self. The body can be seen as an assembly of autonomous organs and this is how the medical model constructs the body. Constipation is often described in terms of 'self';

patients may say 'I'm not my self today', meaning the person or soul is residing in the bowels. Although the bowel and bowel action are part of everybody's everyday experience, such public statements can cause mirth, especially in the media, and can also provide patients with a point of camaraderie.

It is important for practitioners in enterostomal therapy to have a conceptual model using a medical anthropological basis in order to be able to plan care for patients which will enable them to begin to approach their change in body image. Firstly, an adaptation of Lenninger's (1985) sunrise model allows the practitioner to consider all the aspects which influence the individual's path to the health care practitioner to seek the first stage of healing. For the secondary model, use of the nursing process as a framework will be required for assessment, planning, intervention and evaluation of the care given to the individual. By also incorporating Helman's (1991) outline of medical anthropology, an individual care plan may be used to maximise the nurse's knowledge and understanding of the current illness of the individual and helps both individual and nurse to assess how the body image change will impinge on the patient's world. Incorporating these two models into the framework enables the nurse to detach him- or herself from the strict medical frameworks of Western medicine, and allows a deeper understanding of illness and fears. The four areas to be considered are assessment, planning, intervention and evaluation:

Assessment

Questions to be asked are: Why has the individual consented to this particular healing system? What are the individual's feelings on the cause of the problem? What does the individual feel the consequences of the problem to be? What metaphors describe the individual's illness? What rituals might have surrounded this problem? What treatment could be given in the individual's cultural society or group? What other forms of healing would the individual have sought? Do the individual's ideas about the illness concur with the practitioner's ideas?

Planning

Care is planned with the individual, and includes discussion of other agencies which may help and advocacy by the nurse in doctor/patient, patient/ward, patient/environment interactions.

Intervention

Negotiated treatment for the patient is carried out with the involvement of other agreed agencies and healers (e.g. aromatherapy, palliative care, etc.).

Evaluation

Does the individual feel physically healed? How does the psychological adaptation to the body image change the individual? Is the individual able to return to the community to lead a normal and productive life? Has the non-professional idea of illness been discussed and understood?

Disease affects individuals even when it attacks a population, but illness, as well as affecting individuals, frequently affects others, such as family, social network and at times an entire community. In some cultures illness is believed to belong not only to the affected person, but also to the affected person's family, and both are therefore labelled 'ill'.

SEMANTIC NETWORKS

Semantic networks (Fig. 2.1, above) have been described as the way in which people draw upon their beliefs about the causality and significance of their illnesses and the particular treatment options which may be available to them. Good (1977) suggests that there is a 'syndrome of typical experiences', a group of words, experiences and feelings which typically run together for the members of the society. Such a syndrome is not merely a reflection of symptoms linked with each other in natural reality but a set of experiences associated through networks of meaning and social interaction in a society.

Semantic networks produce patterns of association by which they are able to provide for the researcher meanings to elements of medicine. Semantic networks can express emotion in body imagery and constitute it in bodily experience. Networks also enable a framework to be used for understanding the relationship between disease and language. Terminology, folklore and metaphor are all used in semantic networks and make the pathways linking the symbolic to the effective, and language links vocal experience with disease (Turner 1967).

For the Mende people of Sierra Leone, a dirty stomach describes not having had a bowel movement. Diarrhoea causes particular concern to pregnant Mende women, since they believe that the intestine is connected to the uterus, and that diarrhoea will damage the unborn child. For those within the Muslim faith, when a stoma is made above the level of the umbilicus the output is considered to be dirty and defiling and so cannot be touched.

Linguistically the 'bowels' are used by the British to express collected anger. British people are thought not pay much attention to their bodies, and yet have a fixation about their bowels. To have a bowel action every day is for many an almost religious necessity, and the bowel is thought of as the cesspool of the unemptied colon. When British people complain about constipation, they can mean lassitude, headaches or depression. Constipation is defined by many British people as not having their bowels open every day, a belief which harks back to earlier days when it was thought that the intestinal contents putrefy, forming toxins, and leading to the poisoning of the body.

In a small qualitative study using a semi-structured interview, Black (1992) found that the people in the research sample often considered that the individual's cancer or ulcerative colitis was caused by the intestinal contents becoming putrefied, leading to the poisoning of the body. Such beliefs are reflected in British culture, including the theatre and film. In Alan Bennett's film: *A Private Function* a character states that his wife has only two topics of conversation – the royal family and her bowels. In George Bernard Shaw's play *The Doctor's Dilemma*, it is mentioned that the intestine is full of decaying matter and it is suggested that the bowel should be cut out and disposed of, thus releasing the individual from being the centre of infection. In the operation for curing ulcerative colitis the diseased large bowel is removed and within 3 days the individual states how much better he or she feels.

A study by Black (1992), using the illness episode schedule questions, showed the use of semantic networks and explanatory models in descriptions of why the individual had become ill. One person considered his cancer as just retribution for his abuse of his body; some of those questioned believed their illness to be caused by toxins in the air; and one person believed that sitting on toilet seats caused cancer. A common belief among patients with ulcerative colitis was that the disease was caused by a crisis experienced prior to becoming ill. An Asian patient thought that he had let his inner self go and disease had then attacked. After the operation, when discussing his convalescence, he said he would recover by building up his inner self and made a definite

indication that he did not mean by nutrition. A wife considered that the surgeon and enterostomal therapist had caused her husband's cancer because it was the surgeon who had diagnosed it in the first place. She would never afterwards speak to the surgeon or team directly, but only through a third party, and maintained that she hated them for what they had done to her, although it was her husband who had the stoma.

If a framework is to be developed to understand the relationship between disease and language it is important that disease is observed as a socio-historical and cultural phenomenon. Into this network the doctor intervenes diagnostically and therapeutically (Good 1977) and to build a structural theory in body imagery it is important that semantic networks are researched.

Body image is an important part of everyday life and society places an enormous significance on having an attractive body. In a society which sets great value on physical appearance, the ideal body image is one representative of youth, beauty, vigour, intactness and health. There is likely to be a resulting decrease in self-esteem, and an increase in feelings of insecurity, anxiety and unworthiness among those who deviate significantly from this ideal (Smitherman 1981). Shielder's (1935) early description of body image is as a picture we form of our body in our mind. A growing number of complex refinements have since been added to this definition. A look at the literature seems to indicate that our current notion is that it is a perceptual and interpretive and effective experience based upon the body as it physically really is. This experience is dynamic and ever changing in response to alterations in bodily reality (e.g. ageing, trauma). Altered body image exists when individuals experience distress at the nature or at the rate and direction of change of the body and feel that the alteration outstrips their perceived ability to adapt and cope (as with the formation of a stoma). In explanatory models, body image, its norm and abnorm, become referenced against socially learned experiences and against the maturing physiological system of the body. As previously discussed, Wade (1990) also suggests that patients undergoing stoma surgery, who face not only a change in appearance but also a loss of control of elimination, receive a severe blow to their self-esteem and are subject to fears of rejection by friends and relatives and of being ostracised by the society in which they live. The small qualitative study carried out by Black (1992) found that the narratives and interviews showed a clear relationship between opposing elements involved in the individual's change of body image, a contrast between two elements which produces a binary opposition. These oppositions were the basis for constructing the theory of how the individual adapts and changes after such mutilating surgery and copes with body image. 'Before the operation I was a prisoner. I have got my freedom back.' 'I've always been active and now this has stopped me doing anything.' 'I'm an adult in control of my life but when the bag leaks I feel like a baby.' 'Before I would not go out or talk to people at the gate. I thought I would die. Now its wonderful, just like being reborn.' The use of opposites occurs in all discussions with patients with altered body image due to stoma surgery, although they themselves are unaware of how they are expressing emically their meanings of their body change within their own cultural systems. The many binary opposites arising in the patients' narratives and interviews included:

- Internal/external
- In/out
- Self/not self
- Hidden/open
- Control/loss of control
- Private/public
- Inner/outer
- Right/left
- Below/above
- Clean/dirty
- Hot/cold.

The use of binary opposition was very apparent in non-Western individuals undergoing entero-stomal surgery. The Asian patient entering hospital will often have the fear of the prospect of altered body image alongside the rules of social acceptability and taboos of elimination of body waste. People of the Muslim and Hindu faiths consider body waste and elimination to be impure and spiritually polluting, and as such requiring purification by cleansing. Structural anthropology considers that no term is understood in isolation, but is part of a contrasting system built from binary oppositions. Structuralism (Levi-Strauss 1963) holds that the sounds of language impose a logical order on experience in the human mind. The individual classifies perceived phenomena and experiences and uses sound systems as a mental and cultural measure. The suggestion is that in the symbolic realms of culture such as myth and ritual, the human mind uses contrasts and explores contradictions. Bell (1972) considered that 'Man does not see in the way he thinks he sees. Instead of a passive receptive act in which scenes are simply recorded the act of perceiving is one in which man is totally involved and in which he participates actively, screening and structuring.' The internal model of the patient who has undergone entero-stomal surgery is used to create a world of perceived things and events which are mainly learned and largely cultural – what the patient sees is what, through cultural experience, he or she has learned to see.

During the last decade great improvements have been made in the medical care of patients with a stoma, particularly with regard to nursing skills and counselling and the quality of the appliances used. Scientific investigation of patients' psychosocial adjustment has intensified and has been found to give indications for quality of life for these patients. Much of the writing on coping and life events has been undertaken from a sociological point of view (see for example Kelly 1991, Lazarus & Cohen 1982, Black 1990, Bekkers et al 1995, Dietz 1987, McDonald et al 1984). Coping is seen as a central action. It appears that sociological concepts have to be brought into the life event, and if it is conceptualised into a meaningful construction of events, then the model has to extend into the areas of phenomenology and endomethology. In order to understand how an individual copes successfully with a fundamental change, the social action of the model must be examined to uncover the processes which are needed on an individual-centred level.

The way the individual copes with a life event can be compared to an actor giving a performance. When an individual performs he or she is asking observers to take seriously the impression which they are seeing. The performance the individual gives is socialised, moulded and modelled by the particular society in which the individual exists. An individual with a stoma struggles to cope if their private self is an ordinary person with a stoma and their public identity is as someone who is known to have a stoma. The stoma can become a relevant action in some social interactions once the individual's identity as an ostomist is known. The first level of coping is the routine technical skill that is need to keep the unpredictable and incontinent body under control. Under normal circumstances the individual does not usually have to be concerned with these issues, since the person's growth within a culture and society has enabled these functions to be organised into an accepted form. 'Immediately after surgery you have to learn the technological aspect of going to the toilet. You've got to learn a new language, almost a foreign language. There's things you've never seen in your life before, names you've never heard of. Its all strange. Its got to be learned.' Learning to cope with the technical level is learning control of the pollution of the self and the environment and the associated phenomena. These are very private activities, and individuals who are able to cope and manage the body technically can perform before the public audience and appear to be unexceptional. Coping can be conceptualised as an adaptation following illness and the use of cognitive and motor activities employed by the individual to preserve his or her identity compensates for the irreversible impairment.

At the intrasubjective level, however, a person may be able to cope technically, but these skills do not make the threat associated with the stoma disappear – they simply hold it in check. Anger, anxiety and depression are common, and the front presented by the individual, as Goffman (1969) described in his book *The Presentation of Self in Everyday Life*, cannot always hide the undertone of unhappiness: 'It's a nightmare. I wake up at night thinking and worrying about

it. I don't like to dwell in the past but I keep thinking I should've done this, I should've done that. I hate him, the surgeon, for having done this to me. He says, "forget about the past". You can't, its really hard.'

At the interpersonal level of coping, that which has been the private world of the individual now has to become the public world. Some people will know the individual's status and others will not. Managing this knowledge requires sophisticated coping behaviour. The aspects which affect an individual with a stoma are that they have a difference which impinges upon the private self but which does not usually affect the public self. To cope at the interpersonal level, individuals try to recognise the potential for problems and keep their own bodily secrets: 'I felt different. At the hospital it was OK but when I got home and started going out and about again I felt different.' 'Am I going to be able to wear nice clothes again? Will I be able to go on holiday? Am I going to want to go out and meet people and do my shopping?' At these various levels of coping with life events there is often a discrepancy between appearance and reality. There is concealment from the audience of all evidence of dirt and the notion that dirt is looked after in private. In controlling dirt the individual will embody several ideal standards and often these standards are maintained in public by the sacrifice of some of them in private. Often the individual will conceal or underplay activities, facts and motives which are incompatible with the idealised image of the self.

At the intersubjective level of coping, the individual constructs schemas, vocabularies and rhetorics which are used to make sense of what has happened. The use of binary opposites when constructing explanations of how the individual copes then becomes a coping device of its own, with the individual making his or her own semantic networks. Within some social research verbal accounts were common and took the form of scenarios, stories or rationales. In the search for a legitimate identity these vocabularies of coping provided the individual with a framework for reappraising previous events. 'Its never been a problem. We went away for a holiday for a month and I had no problems. I knew I wouldn't. I was confident I could cope. I don't believe there is nothing you can't do. I always say if I could go through all that there can't be anything as bad again.' 'I take each day as it comes. I'm well again and that's great. Its not nice being not normal but I have no regrets. I've got it and that's that. I'm thankful, I couldn't go back to what it was like before.' Verbal accenting appears to be the process by which coping behaviour is initiated to deal with a permanent body change in the individual after enterostomal surgery. Whether the verbal account is a validative description of what has happened to the individual is irrelevant. What is important is that by preserving and presenting a particular version of self within the account, self is then linguistically integrated into a social structure of reality which has been permanently destroyed.

In the attempt to discover the theory and framework used by people who have undergone enterostomal surgery to adapt to their permanent change in body image and identity, it is clear that any discourse concerning the body and body image change will not be complete without considering ideas of shame, anger or guilt related to the illness and to the ultimate body change. The use of the body as a natural symbol demonstrates how the body in health and wholeness offers a model of organic wholeness, while the body in sickness offers a model of social disharmony. Society is only interested in the perfect body, and imperfections – seen or unseen – immediately categorise the person as a marginal member of that particular society.

Clearly, after enterostomal surgery people may feel dirty due to their permanent incontinence, with the bag of faeces or urine on their abdomen acting as a permanent reminder of their un-wholeness and mutilated state. The key word every individual will use in this situation is 'dirt'. Two conditions have been laid down: a set of ordered relations and a contravention of that order. The idea is a system of values which is mutually expressed in given arrangement, for example, defecation on a regular, controlled basis is now violated and permanent incontinence ensues. The individual with a stoma has to

quickly form new schemata and frameworks to be able to return to society and continue to live a normal life. Management of phenomena which are now uncontrolled (noise, smell, sight) have to be learned and incorporated into the individual's existing structures of assumptions. This learning can only take place when the new experience lends itself to assimilation to the existing structure or when the schema of past assumptions is modified to accommodate the unfamiliar. In the early days after enterostomal surgery, people ignore the cues which do not accord with their previous assumption of the control of body function, and learning of self-care can thereby be delayed. Within certain cultures this assimilation and formation of new schemata after enterostomal surgery can be put on permanent hold, since affected individuals will henceforward refuse to have anything to do with the care of themselves. Even within Western societies, negative sanctions and beliefs can be found associated with pollution belief after enterostomal surgery: the belief that gloves should be used to clean oneself; moving out of the partner's bed and room; the establishment of separate washing areas; the use of strong dis-infectants; and in extreme circumstances, giving up work, social and leisure activities and becoming a recluse because the individual considers him-or herself to be dirty and a contaminant. Douglas (1975) maintains that there is no justification for assuming that terror, or even anxiety, is involved in the emotions or beliefs which are associated with pollution, yet from narratives alone we can see that terror and anxiety are among the most frequently used expressions of patients adapting to a new body image. Even if, as Douglas suggests, pollution beliefs are cultural phenomena, the area of enterostomal surgery is one that transgresses all of these beliefs and ideas. In the first few days after a diagnosis of cancer or ulcerative colitis the patient may seek answers to such existential questions as 'Why me? Why now? Why this disease?' – questions which, because of their existential nature, cannot be reduced to biological and material facts. Quickly, these existential questions are replaced by feelings of terror or anxiety concerning the mutilation of the body and the concept of total incontinence. In order to try to answer the existential questions, the individual uses explanatory models to place disease and cure within his or her own framework of understanding.

After enterostomal surgery, how the individual presents him- or herself in everyday life appears to be in the role of an actor, using a dramaturgical approach. This approach allows the individual to give the impression of management and normality to the 'audience', and the individual's status is thereby maintained. The use of cultural and dramaturgical perspectives allows the individual to establish a framework of appearance which must be maintained privately and publicly.

It appears that after enterostomal surgery the individual adopts the strategy of structuralism as a basis to understand the phenomena which will enable the individual to order his or her experiences with regard to the change in body image. It is clear from the narratives that the individual redefines his or her state and can be seen as being at one end of a continuum, not necessarily going from point A to point B. However, it remains to be established whether body image change is brought about around the spatial dimensions of the body, specialised functions of different body regions, or the private and symbolic meanings assigned to body areas by culture. Body attitudes may differ radically in relation to cultural context and it is important to define the role that body image plays in the development and definition of an individual's sense of identity.

3

Quality of life

Quality of life emerges as an important concept and outcome in health and health care practice and a perceived quality of life is an important dimension of the health of both the population in general and of the individual member of that population. The anticipated outcome of stoma care nursing is that it will help patients to an improvement in their quality of life after stoma surgery and the measurement of the patient's quality of life is an important focus in the evaluation of nursing practice. The role that nurses play in assessing and maintaining health will be one of the influences on the quality of life of their patients.

The definition of quality of life is subject to debate and controversy, with sociologists and health researchers divided between those who support a broad concept (Gill & Feinstein 1994) and those who take a more pragmatic view (Guyatt & Cook 1994). There appears, however, to be a general acceptance that there are four domains to be examined when measuring a patient's quality of life. These are the patient's:

- Physical functional status
- Symptoms and side-effects
- Social functioning
- Psychological state.

In measuring quality of life researchers can use generic or specific instruments to provide information. Generic instruments show a summary of health status, functional status and general quality of life, whereas specific instruments will focus on problems to do with a specific disease state, patient group and areas of functioning. The strength of specific indices is that they will focus on the areas of function that are most important to the patient.

Surgical intervention for chronic, congenital or life-threatening illness or trauma of the bowel or bladder results in psychological and physical trauma which impacts on the lives of ostomy patients, either temporarily or permanently. After major surgery, sometimes with little warning, patients suddenly find themselves having to adjust not only to the trauma of surgery, but also to the management of an appliance to enable everyday functioning and excretion, and gradually to continue their lives with an adjusted expectation of normality. Stoma care nurses are key players in the management of stoma patients: they are the first point of contact for patients and provide the education and support that stoma patients need to adjust to their new situation.

Quality of life in stoma patients is the objective in stoma care. Nurses are continually striving to improve their quality of care and need information about the outcome of the care they provide in order to redirect their efforts to areas where the outcome is not ideal. Quality of life assessment can provide them with a quantitative measure of the patient's subjective well-being and functional limitations. The data produced can be considered and used as an indicator of the patient's rehabilitation.

In 1994, a major quality of life international study was set up in sixteen countries using a specific and validated questionnaire. The objectives of the study were:

- To set up a large international study to measure quality of life in stoma patients who are followed by stoma care nurses
- To assess the evolution of the patients' quality of life after surgery over time and to describe this evolution according to country
- To establish the role of the stoma care nurse in the rehabilitation of patients and to allow each stoma care nurse to follow the evolution of his or her patients' quality of life.

The objective at the first stage was to determine the optimum quality of life approach, by means of interviews with patients, stoma care nurses and people who had undertaken research into the well-being and rehabilitation of stoma care patients. The interviews addressed quality of life in depth and also looked at socioeconomic aspects. When the obtained information was evaluated, the optimum quality of life index was sought. This involved looking at the On Line Guide to quality of life Assessment (OLGA, see Appendix) and other databases. When used in conjunction, these systems can offer a comprehensive database of quality of life assessments and their suitable application that will satisfy the context of a proposed study.

In selecting a valid instrument for a quality of life study it is important that the clinical questions are relative to care. The instrument should be:

- Population specific
- Suitable for both cross-sectional and longitudinal studies
- Suitable for measuring appropriate health dimensions
- Suitable for scoring and interpretation by care giver
- Suitable for self-completion by all patients to whom it is administered
- Validated against a generic 'gold standard'.

Patient interviews asked patients how they had been affected by their surgery, about their immediate post surgery life, and about their current daily life, and looked at the social, emotional and physical domains of their life. Opinions of the outcome of surgery varied from realisation of the prolongation of life to rejection of what had taken place. Problems seemed to be more marked in the first few months after surgery. Resocialising varied from patient to patient.

The stoma care nurse interviews looked at patient contact after surgery, problems associated with care, care objectives and suggested improvements. Patient problems, care goals and physical management were easily identified by the nurses, but patients who had reduced their life goals to near reclusiveness were more difficult for the nurse to assess in terms of whether their intervention had had any impact.

The research interviewees felt that the psychological aspects of stoma surgery were often over-emphasised by many researchers in health and social sciences. The following factors played an important part in the patient's ability to make a good recovery:

- Age
- Type and stage of pre-existing disease
- Quality of surgery
- Type of social support
- Personality factors
- Time since surgery.

The interviews demonstrated that a multi-dimensional approach would be appropriate to define the quality of care and to find an instrument that would show the following factors:

- Dimensions of health – physical, psychological and social
- Relative importance at different stages pre- and postoperatively
- Both subjective and objective factors.

In choosing the appropriate quality of life index there was difficulty in finding an instrument that measured functional limitations and the value that stoma patients put on their present health compared to their normal health.

The instrument that appeared to meet the requirements was the Quality of Life Index (QLI) developed by Padilla (1985), which was developed to measure the quality of life as an outcome variable in cancer patients (see also Fig. 3.1). Padilla considered that the problems faced by researchers in investigating the quality of life as an outcome variable were theoretical insufficiency, definitional ambiguity, measurement insensitivity and lack of population norms and fluctuations for targeted ill populations such as patients with cancer.

Using the QLI for the quality of life study, another two sections were added to assess patient satisfaction with medical care and confidence in dealing with the stoma and stoma appliances (see Box 3.1). The questionnaire is self-administered and takes the patient just a few moments to fill

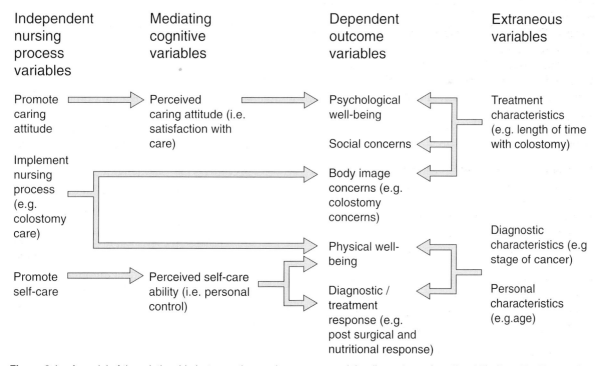

Figure 3.1 A model of the relationship between the nursing process and the dimensions of quality of life (from Padilla 1985)

Box 3.1 Quality of Life questionnaire (Padilla 1985)

Scale	Item number and content
Quality of Life questionnaire	
Psychological well-being (PWB)	9 How much fun do you have? 13 How useful do you feel? 14 How much happiness do you feel? 15 How satisfying is your life? 18 How good is your Quality of Life?
Physical well-being (PHWB)	1 How much strength do you have? 2 Is the amount of time you sleep sufficient? 3 Do you tire easily? 7 How is your present state of health? 11 How much can you work at your tasks?
Body image (BI)	5 Do you feel worried about your stoma? 8 How easy is it to adjust your stoma? 19 How fearful are you of odour or leakage? 22 How difficult is it to look at your stoma?
Pain (PA)	16 How much do you feel pain? 17 How often do you feel pain?
Sexual activity (SXA)	6 Is sexual activity sufficient to meet your needs?
Nutrition (NU)	4 Do you feel your weight is a problem? 10 Do you find eating a pleasure? 12 Is the amount you eat sufficient to meet your needs?
Social concerns (SC)	20 Is the level of contact with your family/friends sufficient to meet your needs? 21 Do you feel rejected by your family and loved ones?
Satisfaction with medical care questionnaire	
Patient satisfaction (PS)	24 I am satisfied with the medical care I receive. 25 When I go for medical care, they are careful to check everything when treating/examining me. 26 The stoma care nurses who take care of me have a genuine interest in me as a person 27 The medical staff who treat me know about the latest medical developments
Improvement (IMP)	28 There are some things about the medical care I receive that could be better.
Experience (EXP)	29 Some of the doctors lack experience with my medical problems.
Self-efficacy questionnaire	
Self-efficacy (SE)	30 How confident are you about cleaning your stoma? 31 How confident are you about changing your appliance? 32 How confident are you about disposing of your appliance? 33 How confident are you about obtaining supplies of your appliance?
Help and advice (ADV)	34 How confident are you about obtaining advice or assistance when necessary?

in. The patient should complete the questionnaire without the assistance of the stoma care nurse. It consists of 34 items in three main sections:

- *Quality of life*: 23 items in seven domains: psychological well-being, physical well-being, body image, pain, sexual activity, nutrition and social concerns
- *Satisfaction*: six items in three domains: patient satisfaction, improvement and experience
- *Self-efficacy*: five items in two domains: self-efficacy, help and advice.

One score is generated per domain, enabling analysis of the results to be performed easily and accurately. From the quality of life related questions a global score is generated called the quality of life index, which gives the best overall information regarding the patient's quality of life. The scores for each domain are 0 for the worst quality of life to 100 for a good quality of life.

The first major analysis, in June 1997, involved the participation of 16 European countries, using patients recruited by stoma care nurses. Each patient completed a questionnaire four times in the first year (at discharge, and at 3, 6 and 12 months). The following year the assessment was on a voluntary basis (one questionnaire at 18 and 24 months). By June 1997, 5289 stoma patients had been recruited postoperatively by 633 stoma care nurses across Europe. At that stage the UK had 117 stoma care nurses participating and had enrolled 1474 patients. Each stoma care nurse across Europe had enrolled a mean of 8.4 patients. The mean age was 61.5 years and male patients were in the majority. The majority of patients had a colostomy and the prime cause was carcinoma.

The European score for psychological well-being was around 60, with the lowest in Portugal and the highest in Belgium. With the global index score the highest again was Belgium and the lowest Portugal.

The evolution of the European QLI, as expected, shows changes with time. The biggest improvement is seen between hospital discharge and 3 months, showing that the patients are generally enjoying a better quality of life. After 3 months the improvement, although continuing, is not so marked.

The relationship with the stoma care nurse after hospital discharge showed that the majority of the patients regarded the stoma care nurse as having a genuine interest in them. These patients had a significantly higher QLI than those who had a poor relationship with the stoma care nurse. Between discharge and 3 month follow-up, analysis showed that if the patient's relationship with the stoma care nurse worsened, the overall QLI score of the patient increased only very slightly. However, where this relationship improved there was a marked increase in the QLI.

In changing appliances most patients had moderate confidence at hospital discharge, but those who were high in confidence were seen to have a higher QLI score. At 3 months, patients who had a decrease in confidence in appliance changing were found to have a decrease in QLI, and likewise the patients who were feeling more confident were experiencing a better QLI. It can thus be seen that helping to increase patients' confidence in changing their appliance will have a beneficial effect on their quality of life.

To date, the results of the European study have shown the questionnaire to be a reliable and acceptable instrument. The scores generally showed improvements after hospital discharge, then a trend for stability over time. Time after hospital discharge is an important factor in the quality of life evolution. The longer the time between the hospital discharge and the first assessment of the questionnaire, the higher the quality of life scores. Time is not the only predictive factor of quality of life evolution after hospital discharge. A close link was observed after hospital discharge and over time between the evolution of quality of life scores and satisfaction with medical care, confidence in changing appliance, or relationship with the stoma care nurse. The more satisfied the patients, the more confident they are, the better the relationships with the nurses, the better the quality of life evolution.

Nurse and patient recruitment continues, with more than 5000 patients enrolled. The importance of the stoma care nurse to the treatment and support of the stoma patient continues to be shown. Interest in individual scores shows areas where quality of life can be improved during patient follow-up (Montreux Study 1998). The study has now been quoted by other medical writers to show the value of specialist nurses to specific patient groups and is the only work available that has been undertaken in any area of nurse specialism to demonstrate their value to a patient group.

4

Medical anthropology

Medical anthropology can be described broadly as the study of cultural beliefs and behaviours associated with the origin, recognition and management of health and illness in different social and cultural groups. It includes issues concerned with 'lay' or 'folk' understandings of the causes and the management of disease and other forms of sickness, and also the more informal systems of health care that exist worldwide, such as treatment by alternative practitioners, folk healers, shamans, etc., as well as those associated with professional Western science based medicine. In addition, it is concerned with issues related to different cultural views of the self in health and disease, as well as shared beliefs, images and practices associated with perceptions of the human body and mind.

The importance of medical anthropology is in the understanding of the cultural context of health and illness. In recent years this has come to be recognised as being of vital importance. As health services in all societies come under increasing scrutiny, the complexity of the relationship between health care and the lifestyles and expectations of populations has become clearer. The ways in which the beliefs and behaviours of populations influence the origin of disease is of increasing importance in the modern world. Such issues need to be studied not only through the large scale quantitative studies of groups of people, but also through the qualitative investigation of patterns of health beliefs and behaviours of such groups. It is often the latter form of research that uncovers the reasons why particular patterns of illness persist or change.

It has become clear that a thorough understanding of people's ways of thinking and acting when ill can lead to insights into many apparently puzzling and strange aspects of health, illness and health care. An anthropological approach will involve a detailed qualitative and ethnographic study of the culture of human groups and the common sets of behaviours which distinguish them from one another in the ways they understand health and illness and how they feel such issues should be managed.

Major social changes have taken place both in industrialised and non industrialised societies. Medical management of patients today involves working with culturally diverse populations and different religions, all with their own attitudes to health, illness and health care. It is therefore important to examine all the factors which may give rise to ill health and influence how it is identified and treated. The issue becomes even more important when conflicts of ideas arise between health professionals, managers and patients about the best ways to manage health sensitively and effectively. In order to provide sensitive care, it is necessary not only to examine the ways in which health care is managed across different cultures, but also to examine it within the various cultural settings. Even those who still favour the Western biomedical model of care cannot have failed to notice that some understanding of the immense variety of local beliefs and practices throughout the world is a prerequisite for the effective management of the health problems of a culturally diverse population. These various perspectives offer a challenge to Western medical approaches to disease.

The patterns of migration between countries and cultures lead not only to anxiety about the geographical spread of disease, but also to concerns about different and conflicting beliefs and practices about health and illness. Medical anthropology is concerned with an unravelling and understanding of these problems. By making the strange familiar, many of the ways of dealing with health and illness which people take for granted can be understood in a new light. In sensitively observing the details of ways in which small groups of people understand health and health care over long periods of time, medical anthropologists attempt to make sense of the ways those in the group perceive and understand the ways in which they live (Gerhardt 1989).

The cornerstone is the ethnographic approach, involving participant observation. It represents a distinct complementary contrast to the quantitative research methods used in much medical and health care research. Medical anthropology allows a reframing of personal practice in the light of a formal understanding of the role of cultural factors. It helps to interpret phenomena involved in health care which otherwise might remain inexplicable, such as why one group considers physical change in their bodies to be a disease while another group does not. It also enables health workers to reflect on their own beliefs as much as on the beliefs of the group they are researching. What we see is entirely conditioned by what we believe is 'normal' and appropriate. For those who work with different social and cultural groups, either in a geographical area or in a community where migration has led to social and cultural diversity, or in a country or society where beliefs and behaviours differ considerably from those of the researchers, medical anthropology helps us to comprehend behaviours and beliefs that differ substantially from our own previous professional and personal experience. Such insights are particularly vital where there are difficulties, or conflicts between professional and family or group beliefs and practices.

Medical anthropology provides a means of focusing attention on a particular domain of interest whilst relating it to the concerns of the discipline as a whole through investigation of religious beliefs and practices, healing systems and the management of misfortune.

Disease process and surgical outcomes

SECTION CONTENTS

5

Bowel cancer

Colorectal cancer is the second commonest malignancy in the Western world. Of the 28 000 new cases in the UK each year, approximately half occur in the rectum. In 1998 there were 14 732 deaths from colorectal cancer in England and Wales (Kocher & Saunders 1999). About 30% of patients present with advanced disease and 25% relapse after complete surgical resection of the tumour. Approximately 50% of patients will either have metastatic disease discovered at surgery or will relapse with metastatic disease (Lederman 1997). The primary treatment for colorectal cancer remains surgery with abdoperineal resection and a permanent colostomy being required for most tumours in the lower rectum. If all cases are included in an analysis of surgery with no additional treatment, the crude tumour free survival of referral of patients is probably as low as 40%, with about 40% dying of uncontrolled disease in the pelvis (Colo News 1997).

The worldwide incidence of colorectal cancer varies 20 fold, with the highest incidence (more than 1000 cases per 100 000 population) seen in Australia and the lowest (fewer than 100 cases per 100 000) in Colombia. Both the large geographic variations in incidence and the observation that population risk changes rapidly on migration – even within one generation – have focused attention on the study of both genetic and environmental factors in the aetiology of bowel cancer. Regional variations in incidence within countries of a similar cultural framework, and the observation that a migrant group's colorectal cancer risk tends towards that of his or her assumed residence, whether higher or lower, implicate environmental and lifestyle factors rather than genetic ones (Cripps 1993). The proportion of truly genetically related colorectal cancers is small, and the above factors already describe the most important lifestyle elements (e.g. dietary). Colorectal cancer risk is thought to be increased by high fat, high meat diets, especially red meat, with contributions also coming from the use of alcohol and tobacco. Some trace elements (e.g. selenium and calcium) may be protective. No occupational influences have so far been identified.

The overwhelming majority of large bowel tumours are adenocarcinomata which have usually arisen from adenomata. The incidence of cancer in polyps is related to size and the degree to which the polyp shows a villous histology. Between 5% and 20% of polyps show either cancer or in situ cancer. It is not known over what time the malignant progression occurs but it is thought to be at least 5 years. Once established, the cancer spreads by local invasion by extension to draining lymph nodes, and by venous embolisation to produce liver and systemic metastases. At diagnosis only 5% of tumours are confined within the bowel wall (known as Dukes' A) and 30–50% have distant metastases (Dukes' C and D), with the remainder in the intermediate (Dukes B) staging. Survival after bowel cancer surgery is directly related to the extent of the tumour at presentation and the aim of screening programmes is to diagnose cancer at the earliest possible stage.

SCREENING

In a screening programme, a test or series of tests is performed on a population that has neither the signs nor the symptoms of the disease being sought, but whose members have some characteristics that identify them as being at risk from that disease, the outcome of which can be improved by early detection and treatment. Screening consists of all the steps that are taken in a programme, from the identification of the population at risk to the diagnosis of the disease. The effectiveness of any screening programme is determined by the sensitivity of the series of tests applied to the population and the effectiveness of the therapy offered to those detected to have the condition.

Getting a screening programme into practice can be a major undertaking, possibly because the programme requires the introduction of a wide range of clinical interventions, with management and information support to ensure quality and to enable audit to be undertaken. The stimulus to screen for colorectal cancer can possibly be due to the lack of impact that modern treatment has had on the long term survival of the patient after diagnosis. Despite advances in treatment and surgical techniques, the 5 year survival rate has been steady for the last 40 years at 35%.

Screening would initially be by the application of a simple, cheap test known as faecal occult test, which would dictate whether the patient needed to go on to a further test. Prior to the haemoccult test the patient is asked to make some dietary restrictions such as large amounts of vitamin C, red meat, and vegetables such as turnips and horseradish for up to 2 days before the test and for 3 days during the testing. The patient takes two pea-sized samples of faeces from the bowel motion which are placed on a test card. Hydrogen peroxide is dropped onto the sample and a colour change is observed. If there is a colour change to blue the test is considered positive and if there is no colour change the test is considered negative. Unfortunately the test is not sensitive enough to know if detected blood is from a tumour or from haemorrhoids. A positive test increases the likelihood of bowel cancer in an asymptomatic well person by approximately 40 times and a negative test reduces that same likelihood by about four times.

Endoscopic screening is the direct viewing of the bowel with an endoscope. To do colonoscopy on large numbers of the population may cause injury and is also expensive. As with all tests and with screening the population at large, compliance is needed, but a different approach is needed for the high-risk groups. Several groups of patients fit this category and these are the patients and families with familial adenomatous polyposis and Gardner's syndromes. These patients have an established autosomal dominant inheritance and a high or absolute cancer risk.

The hereditary non polyposis colorectal cancer syndromes (HNPCC) were recognised by Lynch (Lynch et al 1988), after whom they are named. The Lynch I group is characterised by a preponderance of colon cancers that are site specific in the patient's close relatives. The Lynch II group of patients, as well as having colorectal cancer, will have relatives with carcinoma of the breast, endometrium and ovary; this is known as the cancer family syndrome. Another identified risk factor is a previous personal history of colorectal cancer which gives a 1 in 20 chance of further cancer in 25 years (Mellville et al 1998). (See Fig. 5.1 for distribution of cases of colorectal cancer by site.)

FAMILIAL ADENOMATOUS POLYPOSIS (FAP) (Plate 12)

Familial polyposis has most commonly been known as familial polyposis coli and less commonly as familial adenomatous polyposis coli. As reports of extracolonic manifestations became apparent, it was considered that the term familial polyposis coli was inappropriate. In June 1985, at Leeds Castle in Kent, a meeting of 30 people from 11 countries took place. The meeting's aim was to discuss the care and the problems that arise for those who look after polyposis patients.

The Leeds Castle polyposis group advocated the use of the term familial adenomatous polyposis (FAP), because it describes the nature of the most common intestinal abnormality without implying restriction to the colon.

Diagnosis had previously been made if 100 or more colorectal adenomas were present but this requirement is no longer rigidly applied, especially in patients who have a positive family history. The most important feature of this disease is that one or more adenomas in the large bowel will develop into cancer unless prophylactic measures are undertaken.

The true incidence of FAP is unknown, but an epidemiological study from Denmark estimated a mean annual incidence of 1.3 per million in-

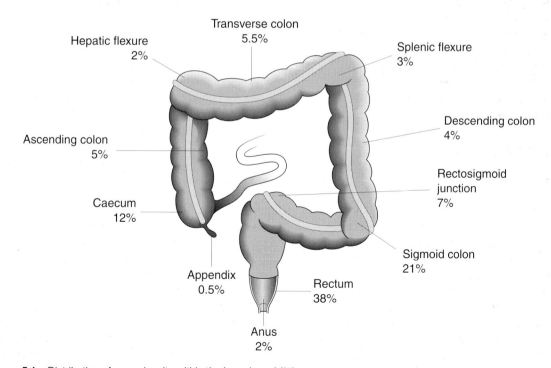

Figure 5.1   Distribution of cases by site within the large bowel (%)

habitants, which equals a birth frequency of approximately 1 in 10 000. This data concurs with information gathered in Sweden and Finland (Bulow et al 1986).

Historically, it is thought that FAP was described by Menzelio in 1721 and Corvisart in 1847. The first definite account was given by Chagelaigue in 1859, describing the disease in a 16-year-old girl and a 21-year-old man. The first familial association was noted by Cripps in 1882 after seeing a 9-year-old boy and his 17-year-old sister (Spigelman & Thompson 1994).

In 1946 Dr Eldon J. Gardner was teaching genetics at the University of Utah and was keen to study hereditary changes. He was told of a family in Utah where nine members had died of colon cancer over three generations. Their average lifespan had been 34 years. During his study of this family, a pattern of cancer emerged known as familial polyposis of the colon, caused by a single autosomal dominant gene. If one parent has the gene, then each of the children has a 50% chance of inheriting the gene.

Other findings during Gardner's study were bony growths, jaw lesions, cysts, fibromas and desmoids. At the time of Gardner's death in 1989, attempts were being made with the use of molecular biology to find the exact location of the gene for FAP. Unfortunately, Dr Gardner did not live long enough to learn that the APC gene was

---

Case study: Sarah

Sarah, aged 27, had been referred to the district general hospital from a hospital 60 miles away with a view to taking over her care and having a surgical formation of an ileal anal pouch. Sarah's diagnosis was FAP. For the last 9 years she had had increasingly worse bouts of diarrhoea and blood loss and ate very sparingly. Sarah was a very scared and anxious young woman with a 3-year-old child. The last thing Sarah wanted was a stoma, and she was definite that she wanted an ileal–anal pouch. Her family history was revealing and quite frightening. Her mother had died in 1993, aged 42, from cancer of the bowel after having had an ileostomy and extensive chemotherapy for FAP. Sarah's uncle (her mother's brother) had a colostomy for FAP. There were two male cousins aged 22 and 25 (her uncle's sons). The 22-year-old had FAP and had an ileostomy and was undergoing chemotherapy. He died while Sarah was in hospital undergoing surgery. The 25-year-old cousin was free of FAP. Sarah's brother, aged 22, had seen Sarah's poor health escalate and had become very disturbed by this and left his job and flat and become itinerant. Sarah was always worried about her brother as he had the same symptoms as she had and she was sure that her brother had FAP. Because of his disturbed state of mind and his upset at the death of his mother he had refused to have a blood test to see if he had FAP.

The year before Sarah's anticipated pouch surgery, she had found a bony growth at the inside edge of her eye in the angle of her nose. It was beginning to obstruct her vision, but to remove the osteoma would have totally disfigured Sarah's face so her head was opened from ear to ear and the osteoma removed that way.

The biopsy notes from her previous hospital showed that there were in excess of 6000 polyps in Sarah's bowel. Sarah was counselled for a one stage ileal–anal pouch construction, but was also told of the other possible outcomes. There would be a chance that a pouch would be constructed but she might have a temporary ileostomy,

or if a pouch could not be constructed there would be a permanent ileostomy, which Sarah was dreading. Sarah was sited for a possible ileostomy in the right iliac fossa.

The surgical outcome was not as hoped or expected. A Dukes' C carcinoma was found in the rectum and another in the sigmoid colon. A panproctocolectomy and ileostomy were done and Sarah's partner, John, was informed. John and his parents were devastated by the news and John did not speak or ask questions of the consultant when told the news. Sarah's recovery was uneventful and she learned to self-care very quickly. She knew that the quicker she coped the sooner she would be able to go home and see her little boy. Sarah confided to the nurse that she was very worried about her son as he had a bony growth on his temple, just like her own. Sarah was referred to the oncology unit for adjuvant therapy and started a long and arduous course of chemotherapy a few weeks later.

The polyposis registry in Newcastle was contacted and information exchanged regarding Sarah's cousin and family. With Sarah's consent the registry at St Mark's Hospital was contacted and she was seen and given support and counselling by them. Sarah was desperate to know if her son had FAP, but the UK policy is not to blood test for chromosome 5 until the child is 10 years old.

It was obvious when Sarah came for chemotherapy that she needed further support and she was referred to the Lynda Jackson Macmillan Centre for Cancer Support and Information. The centre offers help and support for people with cancer, and for those caring for them, via a telephone help line service, drop in information support service, DSS benefits officer, advice and counselling and complementary therapies. The centre was acknowledged as a government Beacon centre, one of eight areas in the UK in 1999, to receive money for the continuation of its work. Sarah understands that her life may be considerably shortened and asks only that she sees her son grow up (Black 1997b).

on chromosome 5. Sarah's case history (above) illustrates only too clearly the genetic inheritance of this disease.

Polyposis registries

The St Mark's Polyposis Register was established in 1925 and became the Polyposis Registry in 1985–6. Within the registry are three groups of patients: those with FAP, those with juvenile polyposis and those with Peutz-Jeghers syndrome. This syndrome describes people who have intestinal polyps and pigmented spots of the mouth, hands and feet. Now that there is recognition of different polyposis syndromes, some families in the registry have been reclassified.

The Thames Regions Polyposis Registry was established in 1992. It was established to bring the demonstrated benefits of a registry to a greater number of health care professionals and covers a large area of south-east England.

The Leeds Castle Polyposis Group was established in 1985 and it aims to coordinate the international efforts that are looking for the aetiology, clinical features, prevention and treatment of FAP in all its manifestations.

EuroFAP was established in 1989 to encourage register formation in countries which do not have them.

Dukes (1952) suggested that:

polyposis is a rare disease and no one surgeon can expect to see more than a few cases in a life time. For this reason it is necessary when studying the disease to collect information from different sources, to collate it, and to keep a register of affected individuals and their relatives.

In the UK there is presently no accurate way of recording how many stomas are raised each year. Estimates are taken from an amalgamation of statistics collected by a hospital research medical company and statistics taken by ostomy companies within the community. These are extrapolated to give an idea of the number of stomas. For many years it has been estimated that there are 100 000 stomas within the UK. This estimate was given by Devlin et al in 1971, and remains as the quoted figure in most articles. A more conservative estimate is that about 60 000 people

Box 5.1 Conditions which may require colostomy formation
• Carcinoma • Diverticular disease • Obstruction • Crohn's disease • Radiation enteritis • Ischaemic bowel • Faecal incontinence • Trauma • Congenital conditions (e.g. Hirschprung's disease and imperforate anus)

in the UK in the 1990s have a stoma of some type. It is thought that there are some 30 000 colostomies at present in the UK, with 7–8000 new cases of colostomy each year. Of these about 5000 will be temporary colostomies.

Colostomy is a temporary or permanent artificial opening made through the abdominal wall into the colon. The site is usually indicated in its description (e.g. a sigmoid colostomy, loop colostomy or transverse colostomy). Conditions which may require a colostomy are listed in Box 5.1 (see also Fig. 5.2).

EVOLUTION OF STOMAS

Pre-Christian Israelites were well aware of the problem of abdominal injuries and the consequences of spillage of 'dirt'. In the Bible (Judges 3, verses 21–23), Eglon, the king of Moab, is stabbed by Ehud: 'he took the dagger and thrust it into his belly and the shaft went in after the blade so that he could not draw the dagger out of his belly and the dirt came out.' Celsus (55BC–AD7), quoted by Dinnick (1934), noted that if the small bowel had been penetrated nothing could be done. However, he felt that if the large bowel could be sutured to the abdomen it would sometimes heal. He noted that occasionally strangulated hernias could break down and form their own abdominal exit or natural stoma and that other types of injuries could lead to traumatic colostomies.

Impediment of the artificial anus or stoma led Lord Chesterfield (1694–1773), cited in Robertson-Smith (1889), to define matter out of

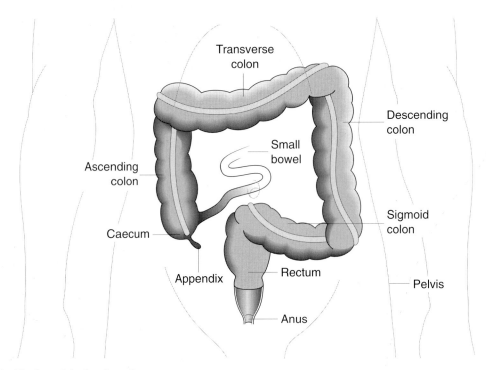

Figure 5.2   The large intestine (bowel)

place as 'dirt' and this word is still used. 'Dirt' implies two conditions: a set of ordered relations and a contravention of their order (Douglas 1966).

The earliest recorded milestone in stoma surgery is the perfection by Heister, in Flanders in 1707, of enterostomy operations on battle casualties. Heister attempted to fix injured gut to the abdominal wall to exteriorise it so that it could not slip back into the peritoneal cavity. He noted that when the wounded intestine had healed, faeces would no longer be voided by the anus but would be excreted by the abdominal wound or stoma. As to wearing a tin or some cloths over the stoma to soak up the excrement, he observed that this was troublesome but 'it is better to part with one of the conveniences of life than to part with life itself' (Heister 1743).

Littré, after dissecting the body of a neonate, observed the imperforate anus and recognised that the rectum was divided into two portions, both of which were closed and connected by only a few strands of tissue. The upper portion of the bowel was filled with meconium and the lower portion was empty. Littré presumed that it would

be possible to bring the upper portion of the bowel to the abdominal surface as a stoma where it would perform the function of an anus (Littré 1732). William Cheselden was said to have been one of the first surgeons to help form a colostomy in 1756. He had noted that some patients with strangulated hernias or congenital malformations developed preternatural exits for the intestinal contents yet continued to live for many years. His patient, Margaret White, had developed an umbilical hernia 23 years previously and at the age of 73 her abdominal wall broke down, allowing the bowel to prolapse from the hernial orifice. Cheselden removed the dead bowel and left the part which was still viable so that a transverse colostomy was raised (Fig. 5.3). Margaret White lived for many years after this procedure, excreting via the colostomy (Cheselden 1784).

Surgeons working on the battlefields (see Figs 5.4 and 5.5) came to realise that if bowel injuries occurred, the dead bowel should be removed and the open bowel pulled through and sutured to the lower end of the wound. This would enable the faeces to pass out of the abdomen in the hope that peritonitis could be prevented, a condition which in those days was fatal. In 1799, at the time of the Napoleonic wars, a French surgeon, Dominic Larrey, organised a surgical service for the assault on Cairo. He expounded that injured bowel should be exteriorised and that in the war situation anastomosis of the bowel should not be undertaken (Larrey 1823), a point which was

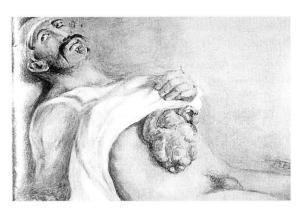

Figure 5.5 Casualty of war

reiterated in 1944 by Ogilvie when undertaking surgery in the Western Desert during the Second World War. Although there were occasional successes in raising stomas, the mortality rate was high as a result of peritonitis caused by faecal contamination. It was not until the second half of the 19th and early 20th centuries that some of the present procedures were developed.

In 1887, Allingham performed a loop colostomy by bringing a loop of bowel onto the abdomen and passing a rod under the loop to prevent it slipping back into the abdominal cavity. A distal and proximal hole was made into the loop of the bowel on either side of the rod. This procedure was used as a diverting procedure and is still popular today (Allingham 1891). Poole (1895) and Von Miculicz (1903) described the exteriorising and excision of a colonic tumour to give a double-barrelled colostomy which could be closed by using a crushing enterotome.

From the middle of the 19th century to the present day the basic concept of colostomy construction has remained unchanged although many technical improvements have taken place. One of these, Hartmann's (1923) elective resection of rectosigmoid cancers with a left iliac-fossa end colostomy, is probably the best-known. The abdoperineal resection for cancer with colicutaneous suturing was introduced by Patey in 1951 and Butler in 1952. The use of colicutaneous suturing and extraperitoneal colostomy helped overcome the problems resulting from stenosis or prolapse of the bowel which had caused many problems with early surgery.

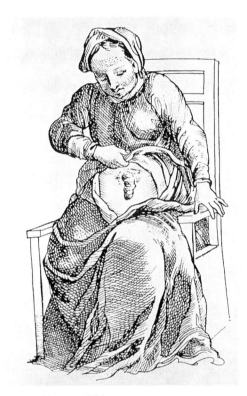

Figure 5.3 Margaret White

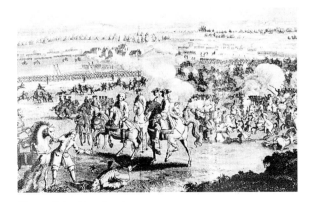

Figure 5.4 Napoleonic wars

Indications

No patient particularly wants to have a stoma, whether permanent or temporary. Most patients will, however, appreciate the advice that one is necessary when the concept of complete and radical clearance of the tumour is explained. Two general indications for an intestinal stoma such as a colostomy are when surgical ablation of the disease requires removal of the anal sphincter and when the surgeon wishes to defunction the bowel owing to the presence of distal pathology or to cover healing anastomosis.

The reasons for a permanent stoma would be due to the removal of the anal sphincter mechanism and could be required under the following circumstances:

- Certain cases of anal cancer
- Low rectal cancer
- Trauma with severe destruction of the pelvic floor area so that reconstruction is impossible
- Functional bowel disease
- Rectal prolapse which cannot be corrected surgically
- Cancer of the rectosigmoid zone, especially if the condition of the patient does not warrant removal of the rectum.

The stoma resulting from these operations would be a permanent one. A permanent colostomy would be constructed from the terminal portion of the intestine and therefore become an 'end stoma'.

Defunctioning the bowel due to distal pathology may be required for the following:

- Perforation
- Fistula
- Trauma
- Intestinal obstruction
- Incontinence
- Functioning bowel disease
- Protection of anastomosis.

The trend over the last 30 years has been away from total rectal excision and in favour of sphincter preserving procedures. This has been made possible by the use of anterior resection and low anastomosis. Technical advances in these areas include hand-sutured colorectal anastomosis and an improved technique for low sphincter resection using the staple gun in which the distal rectum is closed by a transverse stapler.

With the advent of these new procedures it is now technically possible to carry out an anastomosis as distal as is anatomically possible but it has to be decided whether this is justifiable on pathological grounds. If the decision is made to perform an anterior resection and this results in inadequate local clearance of the tumour, it is likely to lead to local recurrence, which would mean the return of the patient for a possible colostomy at that time.

Carcinoma of the anal canal or of the skin at the anal verge (anal margin carcinoma) is quite rare and accounts for only 1–2% of all large bowel carcinomas. This is known as a tumour of the squamous epithelial origin. Regional lymphatic spread here takes place to the inguinal lymph nodes and the pararectal nodes. Here surgery would require a permanent colostomy after an abdoperineal resection operation. This takes the form of total rectal excision with permanent colostomy and can be complicated by delayed perianal healing.

Appliances

Over the last 25 years, mainly thanks to the development of new plastics, much research has gone into designing appliances and in finding the best way to attach them to the skin. Most modern appliances have hypoallergenic barriers to protect the skin and the odour-resistant plastics of the bag ensure they are acceptable to the patient (Plate 13).

The type of appliances used for colostomy patients would be a closed bag which has a filter at the top to let out flatus and charcoal within the filter to help to absorb odour. Postoperatively, until the output from the colon becomes thicker, the type of bag used will be a drainable bag. In the initial days postoperatively this is cared for by the nursing staff but later patients are gradually introduced to the concept of self-care. Although the colostomy bag will ultimately be a closed appliance with a filter, thought must be given to the type of appliance that will suit different patients' needs and enable them to perform their everyday activities. Assessment of the whole patient is important: one must take note of the person's way of life, lifestyle, disabilities, sight, poor faculties, arthritis, and any other possible problems that are seen when looking after the colostomy patient (see Ch. 9 on stoma appliances).

The first appliance is chosen by the nursing staff or the stoma therapist, having assessed the needs of the patient preoperatively and post-operatively. Later, as patients adjust to the surgery and their colostomy, they will become aware that there are other bags on the market which they might like to look at. It takes time for patients to get used to a new way of life. Later, when more settled, patients may want to see other appliances. Samples can be obtained from the ostomy companies and patients can meet the companies at patient open days. In the early days in hospital a clear bag is invariably used so that the stoma and output can be observed until the patient has settled down and is able to start caring for him- or herself. Many older patients prefer to stay on a transparent bag because it enables them to see themselves applying the bag when doing their own procedure at home and looking into a mirror. For patients who do not wish to see the contents of their stoma output, opaque bags are available (see Figs 5.6 and 5.7). Most bags will come in clear or opaque with ready-cut holes to fit in a one- or two-piece appliance.

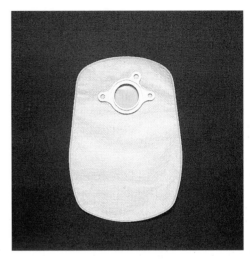

Figure 5.7   Two-piece colostomy bag

SURGICAL PROCEDURES
Colostomy

Colostomies may be raised as a temporary or as a permanent stoma depending on the circumstances leading to surgery (Fig. 5.8) (see also Plate 14).

Temporary colostomy

A temporary stoma may be raised to allow the bowel to heal. The faecal output is diverted. This is done if the surgeon feels that in joining the bowel at this stage, or allowing continuity of faecal flow, there may be contamination of the new surgical area. Likewise, when the peristalsis of the bowel starts again there may be tension on the new anastomosed bowel. A temporary defunctioning stoma may also be raised on patients who have distal obstruction that has perforated from benign or malignant lesions including diverticular disease or traumatic injury (Rutegard & Dahlgren 1987). A temporary stoma may also be raised to cover anal surgery such as the gracilis operation, or to cover plastic surgery such as grafts to pressure sores. When the intention is to defunction the bowel for longer than the anticipated 3–6 months, it is better for patient management to have an end stoma constructed as opposed to a loop colostomy or ileostomy. While an end stoma is easier to care

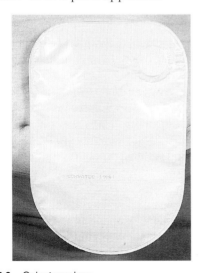

Figure 5.6   Colostomy bag

for from the patient management point of view, reversal requires major surgery again. A defunctioning loop stoma, while easy to construct and reverse, may not fully defunction the bowel.

It is estimated that there may be 7000–7500 people in the UK with temporary stomas that are created each year (Stringer 1985, Fleming 1984). New surgical techniques such as the neo sphincter and the ileal–anal pouch will require the formation of a temporary stoma. As more and more surgeons are finding that these operations are becoming easier to do in district general hospitals, the formation of temporary stomas is likely to increase (Allison 1995).

A transverse loop colostomy is commonly placed in the upper right quadrant of the abdomen, a location which may cause management problems for the patient who has pendulous breasts or a low rib cage, and cause difficulty when sitting and bending. This area is likely to be the patient's natural waistline and difficulty is experienced with clothes and belts. Finding a suitable appliance may also be a problem as the difficult positioning of the stoma may lead to leakage. It is estimated that 20% of transverse stomas will prolapse causing further management problems for the patient, and a further 20% will have a peristomal hernia. For the loop stoma, the biggest problem is the stoma prolapsing. Data collected by Nasmyth (1984) indicated that there are more management problems with transverse colostomies and that there were more odour problems. Nordstrum & Hulten (1987) found that in a group of patients with a mean age of 70 years with transverse loop colostomies, 34% had a prolapsed stoma and 67% had a parastomal hernia.

Reversal times of temporary stomas depend on the surgeon and his or her policy. In some units the reversal time is as little as 1 month following initial surgery if investigations have shown the anastomosis to be healed. To attempt closure sooner than this after primary surgery is a risk and often the patient has not had time to make a reasonable recovery.

Realistically, in most district general hospitals, the turn around time of reversing a stoma is between 3 and 6 months. Sometimes, for whatever reason, the occasional patient falls through the net and remains with a temporary stoma for a few years. Patients often come to outpatient appointments several months after initial surgery and are told by the doctor that they can go onto the waiting list to have their stoma reversed, only to say that they are happy to live with the stoma. The doctor may become quite confused, having assumed that reversal of the stoma is what the patient would want. Strangely enough, patients with a Hartmann's procedure that can be reversed often decide to keep the stoma because they reason that they will be clean and not have problems with re-learning continence, or with potential incontinence. As many as 47% of patients do not have their temporary stomas reversed, either through their own choice or because of surgical difficulty.

There is a recognised morbidity associated with the reversal of temporary stomas and it is not unusual to find faecal fistulas, sepsis or abscess formation. The formation of a temporary loop ileostomy is felt to be a better option than a temporary transverse loop colostomy as it is located in the right iliac fossa and management may be easier for the patient with a better selection of appliances available.

Doctors often feel that if they can tell a patient that the stoma is temporary and will be reversed in 6 weeks, then the patient will accept the situation. Unfortunately, some patients rely on every word the doctor tells them and this can cause conflict because the stoma care nurse knows that realistically the reversal time at his or her hospital is between 12 and 24 weeks. By adopting the stance that the patient is told that the stoma is permanent until it is reversed when the healing process is completed, patients can go home and adapt to their lives with a stoma without having an expected time for the reversal of the stoma in mind and becoming depressed when they are not admitted to the hospital on that very day.

End colostomy (see Fig. 5.12)

An end colostomy is raised after total rectal excision, as in an abdominoperineal resection (see Fig. 5.9). The bowel is brought through the abdominal wall and the colon is sutured to the skin using dissolvable sutures. There should not be tension on the bowel as it comes through the skin as this can lead to retraction.

The stoma is sited in the left iliac fossa and should protrude at least 1 cm above skin level. The end colostomy is also used following a Hartmann's procedure (Fig. 5.10), when the rectal stump is oversewn. End stomas can be managed with an appliance, a plug or by irrigation (see Ch. 9 on stoma appliances).

Loop sigmoid colostomy (Fig. 5.11)

The sigmoid colon is mobilised and the loop of colon exteriorised and the abdomen closed. A rod or bridge supports the bowel and the bowel is opened longitudinally and mucocutaneous

sutures are inserted. The loop transverse colostomy employs a similar procedure and the stoma is in the right upper quadrant.

Divided (Devine) colostomy

This procedure is carried out where it is important to avoid any faecal contamination of the defunctioning end of the bowel. The bowel is divided and both ends are brought out onto the abdominal wall. The proximal end is the output bowel stoma and the distal end is a mucous fistula. The two stomas should be some distance from each other to allow non-leakable pouching and easy management that patients can do on their own. Unfortunately, mucous fistulas are often placed at the end, middle or top of the suture line, causing difficulties in management.

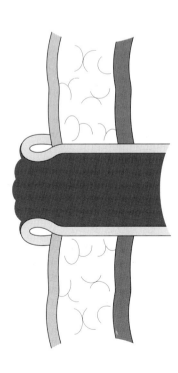

Figure 5.8   Stoma cross-section

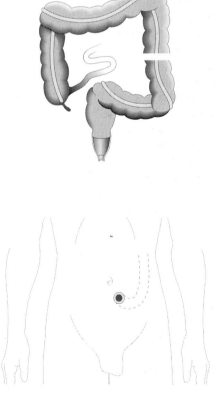

Figure 5.9   Abdominoperineal resection

Ascending colostomy

This (comparatively unusual) colostomy will be placed in the right iliac fossa. The output is very much like the output from an ileostomy. The ascending colostomy will relieve problems in the transverse bowel and onwards to the descending bowel.

The electrically stimulated neo-anal sphincter

For some patients the thought of going through the rest of their lives with a colostomy is abhorrent, and they will do anything to avoid it. With continual innovations and improvements in surgery, for some patients there is now the possibility of reconstruction of the anal sphincter. These advances in colorectal surgery have been

pioneered at the Royal London Hospital and at Maastricht, in the Netherlands. Outcomes to date have been encouraging.

Patients who suit the criteria for this operation fall into three groups:

- Those with faecal incontinence where previous surgery has failed to restore continence
- Those where the sphincter mechanism has to be removed, as in low rectal cancer
- Congenital absence of sphincter mechanism.

The main procedure involves the transferring of the gracilis muscle from the inner thigh. This is tunnelled under the skin and wrapped around the anal canal in a gamma configuration. Prior to this the gracilis has to be prepared for the operation by vascular delay allowing an improved vascularity and viability of the muscle after transposition. At this time a loop colostomy is

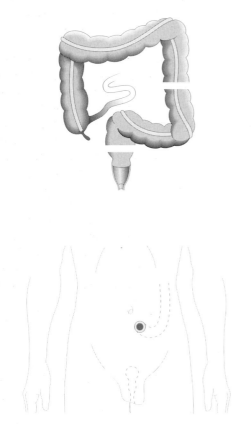

Figure 5.10 Hartmann's procedure

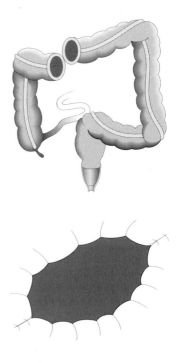

Figure 5.11 Loop colostomy

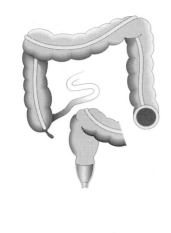

Figure 5.12   End colostomy

raised to ensure the faecal output is diverted while healing takes place. If possible, the defunctioning loop stoma is raised through a laparoscopic technique.

Electrical stimulation takes place via small electrodes that are stitched into place on the nerve of the gracilis muscle and connected by a wire under the skin to the electrical stimulator which is placed just below the ribcage in a pocket of fat.

Stimulation is usually started at about 10–12 days postoperatively. This is needed as the gracilis muscle is a type 2 fast twitch muscle which has little tone and rapidly tires when made to work. The gracilis has to be pro- grammed to become a fatigue resistant, type 1 muscle, able to maintain tone. Stimulation of the muscle is by the implanted stimulator which is controlled by a hand-held magnet.

Closure of the stoma is done at about 3 months after stage 2. Once bowel function has started, the patient is taught to operate the stimulator using the magnet (Stuchfield et al 1997).

The patient, once recovered, can return to daily activities, but because there is an implanted electric stimulator some care has to be taken. The stimulator will show up at airport security checks and patients are issued with a card explaining that there is an implanted electrical stimulator. Other electrical hazards such as large stereo speakers, generators and power lines may switch off the stimulator.

Success in this operation is likely for patients who are well motivated and well selected. Patients will need family support through several operations and recovery.

ODOUR AND FLATUS

Probably the biggest worry of patients with stomas is whether they will produce an odour detectable by other people. Reassurance should be given that appliances today are made of excellent, technologically refined plastics and are one use only. If the appliance becomes detached or leaks there will be odour, but as long as the appliance is properly attached and sealed all the way round there will be no odour.

The appliance would usually be changed in the bathroom/toilet, where people normally go to open their bowels, and at this point there will be odour. Using a supermarket air freshener will mask the smell, but can sometimes be equally unpleasant. Alternatively, patients are now able to buy products like air fresheners, but which are actually absorbers, and these act chemically upon the odour without leaving an unpleasant smell. The cheapest and easiest way is to strike a match when the appliance is emptied and throw the lighted match down the toilet pan. This effectively burns the gas and eliminates the smell.

Colostomy appliances all have very efficient filters on them and they serve two purposes. In the filter there is a black ring of charcoal that helps to absorb and dissipate odour. The second purpose is to let flatus out of the appliance to stop ballooning of the bag.

If necessary, there are special drops and powders that can go into the appliance to help with odour. All these are on prescription, but add vastly to the GP's expenditure, and other than in severe circumstances are not essential items. Discussion with the patient on dietary intake may help to combat some particularly unpleasant odours (see Ch. 23).

Flatus may cause problems for patients. However, there are now colostomy appliances with very effective flatus filters that stop the appliance ballooning, and in the last 2 years ileostomy appliances with effective flatus filters have become available. Flatus in an ileostomy appliance used to be a problem, as the appliance had to be undone at the bottom to allow the flatus to be expelled. This meant that the patient had to find a toilet, which was not always easy.

Technology from the ostomy industry produced a filter that did not block in wet circumstances and allowed flatus to be dispelled, so giving many patients a better quality of life.

Yoghurt and buttermilk are useful components of meals since they help to reduce flatus and odour. They are particularly useful when patients are on antibiotic therapy. Undisciplined eating patterns will give rise to problems such as irregular gut action and excessive flatus with the need to change or empty the appliance more often (see also Ch. 23).

6

Inflammatory bowel disease: ulcerative colitis and Crohn's disease

The term inflammatory bowel disease covers two main diseases, namely ulcerative colitis and Crohn's disease. Inflammatory bowel disease can occur against a background of various genetic and environmental influences. Ulcerative colitis and Crohn's disease are seen within families. Patients with families who have colitis are more likely to see other relatives with colitis. Ashkenazi Jews are more prone to inflammatory bowel disease than non-Jews. People of European origin are more susceptible than people of indigenous or Oriental origin. Within China, for example, ulcerative colitis is particularly rare. Studies that have looked at the increase in the frequency of inflammatory bowel disease among South African and American black populations have indicated that environment is a factor.

Both diseases exhibit periods of remission and relapse. Many patients suffer severe discomfort. A lot of the research on the incidence of Crohn's and ulcerative colitis is from populations that have a comprehensive health care system, mostly northern Europeans and white Americans (McConnell et al 1986).

Variability in the incidence rates of ulcerative colitis may reflect different attitudes to the inclusion of degrees of proctitis. Low disease frequencies are seen in southern Europe and in tropical areas but it can often be confused with infective diarrhoeas such as *Shigella* dysentery, etc. The gender difference is small, with women appearing to be affected slightly more often than men in both Crohn's disease and ulcerative colitis.

Although ulcerative colitis may be diagnosed at any age, it is most commonly diagnosed in early adulthood, with secondary and tertiary peaks of the disease being reported in the elderly. This may be non-specific inflammatory disease or antibiotic induced colitis. With ulcerative colitis, which affects between 50 and 150 per million of the population, females are affected slightly more often than males. Crohn's disease affects between 20 and 90 persons per 100 000 in Europe and the USA. Geographical variation is seen more in Crohn's disease than in ulcerative colitis. The peak incidence of Crohn's disease occurs between the 2nd and 4th decades, with the distribution being equal between male and female.

PREDISPOSING FACTORS

Statistically, it has been difficult to show whether rising incidence rates of Crohn's disease and ulcerative colitis are due to diagnostic transfer between the two diseases or an increased awareness by clinicians of symptoms and more sophisticated investigations. No occupational difference or social class differences have been reported, but a slight elevation in the incidence of Crohn's disease is seen in white-collar workers. Other predisposing factors in Crohn's disease and ulcerative colitis may be dietary. There is consistent evidence to suggest that patients with Crohn's disease have a higher sugar intake in their diet than do people studied as a control (Langman 1990). With ulcerative colitis, it is thought by many that the removal of dairy products from the diet may help and cause remission in disease.

Infection

It is thought that both Crohn's disease and ulcerative colitis may have an initial base of disease or infection or an infected illness, but as yet no supporting evidence for this has been found.

Childhood factors

Bergstrand & Hellers (1983) found that lack of breast-feeding may predispose to Crohn's disease but current data is not totally convincing. For both Crohn's disease and ulcerative colitis no other childhood predisposing factors have come to light.

Drugs and the risk of disease

The use of the oral contraceptive pill has been associated with Crohn's disease and ulcerative colitis, but again the basis of this is uncertain (Vessey et al 1986). Likewise, the use of non-steroidal anti-inflammatory drugs has also been associated with Crohn's disease, ulcerative colitis, colonic haemorrhage and perforation, but not with the actual onset of chronic inflammatory bowel disease. In one study (Rampton et al 1983), however, an association was found between the use of paracetamol and the exacerbation of colitis.

Smoking

As with other conditions, inflammatory bowel disease has a relationship with cigarette smoking, but in inflammatory bowel disease the relationship is unique in that while Crohn's disease appears to be made worse by smoking, ulcerative colitis appears to improve. Although it is not clear why this remarkable difference exists it does have an important implication for possible treatment strategies and directions for future research (Osborne & Stansby 1994). Samuelson (1976) first reported the relationship between ulcerative colitis and smoking. He found that patients with ulcerative colitis were less likely to be smokers than the general population. In 1982 Harries et al confirmed the significance of these observations. Since then the relationship between smoking and ulcerative colitis has been repeatedly found by others, with evidence that there is a dose related effect: people who smoke fewer than 25 cigarettes per day are as likely (within a 10–20% range) to get ulcerative colitis as non-smokers (Franceschi et al 1987).

Whether a difference between males and females in ulcerative colitis and smoking exists is not clear. Some studies have shown the negative effect of smoking on ulcerative colitis to be greater in women who are current smokers whilst other studies have failed to show a significant gender difference. It has been suggested that the fall in the number of current smokers in recent years may explain the increasing incidence of ulcerative colitis that has been reported over a similar time period (Tysk & Jarnerot 1992).

Some studies have suggested there could be a rebound effect in giving up smoking before the development of the disease. Smokers who give up may be more prone to develop ulcerative colitis than people who have never smoked. In a study by Motley et al (1987), it was shown that 52% of patients with ulcerative colitis developed the disease within 3 years of stopping smoking. Pullan (1994) suggests that the use of nicotine gum or transdermal patches may help people with active ulcerative colitis, having a therapeutic effect on the disease without exposing the patient to some of the detrimental effects of smoking.

Crohn's disease and smoking

Far less is known about the role of smoking and Crohn's disease, although the study by Harries et al (1982) which demonstrated the relationship between smoking and ulcerative colitis failed to show such a relationship for Crohn's disease. When an age and sex match control study was carried out, patients with Crohn's disease were found to be more likely to be smokers than the controls. Similar increases have since been shown in several other studies. A study by Pearson (1990), in which 184 patients with Crohn's disease were asked about current and previous smoking habits as well as previous exposure to tobacco smoke when aged 0–15 years, confirmed the findings of an increased risk in smokers, with the relative risks being 1.5% for men and 5% for women. The risks of developing Crohn's disease were 1.16% for men and 2.5% for women if they had been exposed to regular passive smoking as a child.

It therefore appears that smoking increases the risk for Crohn's disease sufferers and decreases the risk in ulcerative colitis. Any attempts to explain this relationship have been complicated by the fact that the causes of both diseases remain unknown. Some doctors are not aware of this complex relationship and patients may receive contradictory advice.

Because health education is thought to play a significant role in preventive medicine, few physicians could countenance suggesting that patients with ulcerative colitis should start smoking. A far stronger case can be made by physicians and clinicians that patients suffering from Crohn's disease should attempt to give up smoking. Perhaps, ultimately, understanding why smoking has such an effect in inflammatory bowel disease – both in Crohn's disease and in ulcerative colitis – may help to lead to advances in the understanding of the disease as a whole.

ULCERATIVE COLITIS

Management

Medical management

Although, as previously discussed, the aetiology of ulcerative colitis remains obscure, improvements have been made in its management and in the use of drug therapy. The use of colonoscopy has made a major impact on management in demonstrating the severity and extent of the disease and for long-term monitoring. Examination of the biopsy samples can detect changes. These include the potential change to malignant disease, which can have implications for management. Medical and surgical cooperation can only prove beneficial for patients.

Diagnosis

In ulcerative colitis diagnosis is usually straightforward and can be made upon taking of a history of the gradual worsening of diarrhoea with the passage of blood and mucus but with little pain. Sometimes patients present with a short history of severe diarrhoea and bleeding and with marked systemic changes. The diagnosis can often be confirmed at the patient's first visit to the outpatient clinic, by undertaking a sigmoidoscopy. At this procedure biopsies will be taken even if the mucosa appears to be normal, as histological changes can still indicate inflammatory bowel disease.

> **Box 6.1**   Possible causes of diarrhoea with blood
>
> - Ulcerative colitis
> - Crohn's disease
> - Ischaemic colitis
> - Carcinoma – villous adenoma
> - *Shigella* dysentery
> - *Clostridium difficile*
> - Amoebic dysentery
> - *Campylobacter coli*

It is also important at this stage to exclude other possible causes of diarrhoea with blood (see Box 6.1).

Diagnostic investigations for ulcerative colitis and Crohn's disease (see also Box 6.4, below)

Sigmoidoscopy. Sigmoidoscopy can be undertaken at the patient's first visit to clinic with little discomfort for the patient and no preparation needed. Here a diagnosis of proctitis or procto-colitis can often be made, especially if a biopsy is taken. With rigid sigmoidoscopy there is only a limited view and it can be obscured by stool. Often the sigmoidoscope can only go as far as 20 cm since outpatients have usually not been previously prepared with bowel preparation.

Flexible sigmoidoscopy. With this procedure it is possible to examine the whole of the sigmoid colon and some of the descending colon to the level of the splenic flexure. This procedure can also be performed on an outpatient who has come to the clinic and who has had limited bowel preparation, with or without a disposable enema during the clinic visit. This procedure will often be undertaken in the endoscopy clinic with the patient coming in as a day-care patient. Flexible sigmoidoscopy will give additional information to that which has been gained by rigid sigmoidoscopy.

Barium enema. As fibre optic endoscopy becomes more and more widely used, the use of barium enema will have small value as an initial procedure in ulcerative colitis. It will remain useful in helping in a differential diagnosis between Crohn's disease and ulcerative colitis and also in those patients for whom it is not possible to perform flexible endoscopy (for example where the patient experiences pain or where there are technical difficulties). Generally, with barium enema it would be difficult to detect mucosal disease but it would be possible to detect strictures and any small carcinomas. Because of recent advances in endoscopic examination less reliance is now placed on X-ray studies such as barium enemas as patients are managed by the specialist colorectal team.

Colonoscopy. Colonoscopy is valuable in the management of ulcerative colitis, in the determination of the extent of the inflammatory bowel disease and in regular screening for patients with long-term colitis. Colonoscopy enables the clinician to see the whole of the large bowel. Colonoscopy also plays an important part in the management of patients with colitis in screening for any changes from colitis to carcinoma. This is an important consideration which may influence the long-term management of the disease.

To undergo colonoscopy the patient requires bowel preparation and usually some form of sedation and/or analgesia. Again, the procedure can be carried out in an endoscopy unit on a day-care basis. For most patients who undergo a colonoscopy procedure, valuable information is gained as to the extent of the disease. If the procedure is carried out by well-trained clinicians or specialist nurses it causes minimal discomfort.

Treatment

Substantial benefits are gained for patients who are involved with a team of good clinicians and surgeons in the treatment of their inflammatory bowel disease. In many areas physicians can feel that surgeons operate too soon on patients with ulcerative colitis and likewise surgeons often level criticism at physicians for leaving the patient too long in referral for surgery. Where there is good cooperation on a regular basis, and each physician and surgeon understands and works with the other, the patient can only benefit.

Relapse (Box 6.2)

Assessment

In the treatment of an acute relapse in ulcerative colitis the appropriate decision has to be made quickly. For some an operation may be inappropriate, but in other cases the patient may die if an operation is delayed too long. Daily consultations as to the state of the patient's health should be part of his or her care.

Mild relapses can be managed at home and many patients know how to look after themselves and when to seek hospital advice. Severe relapses will need hospital treatment. Such patients will have an overall systemic change – possibly anaemia, tachycardia, pyrexia, sweating, anorexia and nausea. There is often dehydration with electrolyte imbalance, especially if diarrhoea has been persistent. Rectal bleeding with the diarrhoea may be severe.

Treatment (Box 6.3)

The aim of treatment during a relapse is to enable the patient to go into a remission and to be discharged from hospital. There are particular dangers at this stage of acute toxic dilatation and perforation of the bowel. When a patient is admitted with a severe relapse from ulcerative colitis, there are three main aims of treatment: resuscitation, therapeutic intervention and observation. Intravenous fluids will be required for rehydration and the correction of electrolyte imbalance. If the patient has been bleeding rectally, blood transfusion may be necessary. With immediate resuscitation treatment, patients often respond quickly, and symptoms begin to ease within 24–48 hours, but a total remission may take somewhat longer.

In the early days of admission particular attention should be paid to the size of the abdomen – measuring the abdominal girth can give useful information.

The reason for emergency surgery such as colectomy within the first 2 or 3 days of a relapse is dilatation of the bowel and continuing symptoms. It is at this stage of the severe relapse (or several relapses) that referral to the surgical team may be made. Emergency surgery results in an unprepared, ill patient who is unable to benefit from elective surgery with proper counselling pre- and postoperatively, and who has no time to gain an understanding of the choices of surgical options. It is known that patients who undergo surgery with good preoperative counselling make far better recoveries (Black 1994d).

Remission

When the patient is in remission, the aim of management is to prevent any relapse and should include regular monitoring, drug treatment and dietary help and advice. It is not thought that a specific dietary factor is responsible for colitis although many people find dietary manipulations help them and many will opt to remove milk and other dairy products from their diet. Although the exclusion of specific foods has not been proved to be of benefit, patients who feel that the absence of certain foods in their diet helps to keep them in remission should be encouraged to continue. It is considered that a high residue diet can help to form and produce a soft formed stool and also reduces the possibility of constipation. Many patients with ulcerative colitis

---

Box 6.2 Signs of acute relapse in ulcerative colitis

- Tachycardia
- Fever
- Anaemia
- Abdominal pain and tenderness
- Vomiting and nausea
- Abdominal distension

Box 6.3 Main points of management for acute relapse of ulcerative colitis

- Correct anaemia (possible blood transfusion)
- Intravenous fluids with electrolyte correction
- Exclude infections
- Systemic steroid administration
- Continual observation
- Abdominal measurement and abdominal X-ray if abdominal distension is present

cannot tolerate green vegetables or fresh fruit or anything with a skin and very little (if any) bran in their diet. It is more a case of advising the patient on the correct dietary intake to give them the correct vitamin and nutrient level, taking into account what suits them and gives them a reasonable quality of life at that time.

Drugs

It appears that sulphasalazine is the drug with proven value in the maintenance of remission for patients with ulcerative colitis. The usual dose is 1 g twice daily but for some patients 4 g a day may be prescribed. Side-effects of this drug are nausea and vomiting, and abdominal discomfort. The more toxic effects in some patients can be haemolytic anaemia or bone marrow suppression and the patient must be closely monitored.

It has been observed that in the male patient sulphasalazine can cause suppression of sperm, resulting in male infertility, but apparently this can be reversed on stopping treatment with sulphasalazine (Turnburg 1989).

The apparent therapeutic efficacy of sulphasalazine lies in 5-aminosalicylic acid, otherwise known as 5-ASA. It is thought that encapsulated forms of 5-ASA which can release their contents into the large bowel are less troublesome, and trials of mesalazine (encapsulated 5-ASA) and Dipentum®, which is two 5-ASA molecules linked together, suggest that they are equally as good as sulphasalazine, but have fewer side-effects.

Early treatment to stop a relapse can be helped by administering topical steroids and these come in the form of the Predsol® enema which can be administered by the patient every night for about 10 days and can help in inducing a remission. Most patients can manage to administer these themselves at home and retain the enema in their rectum overnight. Another form of topical steroid administration is Colifoam® but this does not go into the bowel as high as a liquid enema.

Patients with ulcerative colitis who do not require hospitalisation may nevertheless have persistent symptoms which interfere with their life, work, social activities and well-being. The disease also has an effect upon families. Continual application of sulphasalazine and systemic and rectal steroids may help but only for a limited time. Often with this group of patients (who may have frequent relapses running into one long relapse), anaemia occurs. Patients by this time may well have been motivated towards the consideration of surgery, either by their gastrointestinal physician or, more generally, by their continual ill health which is preventing them from leading a normal life. It will be at this stage, when there is referral to the surgeons, that the stoma care nurse will be asked to discuss with the patient the possibility of surgery and the options that are now available. This meeting may take place on the ward, or it may be in the outpatient department or in the patient's home.

One of the considerations of surgery – apart from the fact that it can improve health generally and very quickly – is that a patient who has had colitis for more than 10 years may become liable to develop carcinoma of the colon. Susceptibility to carcinoma of the colon increases each decade after the 10th year of the onset of ulcerative colitis, particularly in those who have had the disease diagnosed at a young age and who have had continual symptoms. Rectal biopsies in these patients which show no signs of dysplasia can probably exclude a colorectal cancer, but detection of dysplastic changes is a strong indicator that the patient would benefit from colectomy to prevent the development of colorectal cancer.

Patients with ulcerative colitis should have a colonoscopy performed every two years if they are asymptomatic but more frequently in those with symptoms. This form of screening appears to offer a reasonable chance of preventing colorectal cancer in susceptible individuals.

Complications of ulcerative colitis

One of the extracolonic manifestations of inflammatory bowel disease is pyoderma gangrenosum (Turnburg 1989). This skin disease can complicate a relapse of ulcerative colitis, but tends to improve as the bowel disease is treated. Colectomy in itself will not cure pyoderma gangrenosum. It is at this stage that corticosteroids are most beneficial for patients showing the signs of this systemic upset, and usually the disease improves promptly once therapy has started. Other forms of immunosuppressive therapy (e.g. azathioprine or 6 mercaptopurine) may be needed for patients with severe cases of pyoderma gangrenosum.

Joint disease (Turnburg 1989) is often seen as a complication of ulcerative colitis. After surgery and the cessation of steroids patients may find that they have arthritis, and in some cases attacks can be very severe. The large joints (knees, hips, shoulders, and often ankles) are most often affected, and the arthritis tends to follow the course of the bowel disease. Treatment for the bowel disease in the form of steroids can help the joint symptoms, but once surgery has been performed and a colectomy has been undertaken, steroids are reduced or finished and many patients then complain of various degrees of joint pain. In these cases drugs such as the non-steroidal analgesics are helpful and aspirin may be used. However, while the patient has ulcerative colitis the use of aspirin can worsen the colitis.

Proctitis

In some patients with ulcerative colitis the disease does not extend beyond the sigmoid colon and is limited to the rectal area. These patients usually progress well and do not develop the other side-effects of ulcerative colitis. The manifestations of ulcerative colitis in these patients are generally less severe and often well controlled topically. Again, with these patients topical treatment by Predsol® enema or Colifoam® is often very helpful and is all that may be needed. Sometimes treatment with sulphasalazine together with a high residue diet can help (Turnburg 1989).

CROHN'S DISEASE
Diagnosis

The diagnosis of Crohn's disease can often be delayed, and patients may have seen several doctors before the correct diagnosis is given. Symptoms are non-specific and variable. Many of these patients require life-long management and advice. Patients with Crohn's disease often do not require surgery, but a good relationship is needed between the gastroenterologist and the patient. The disease is often well established before there is any confirmation of diagnosis, which is usually dependent on a combination of clinical and investigative features that make up a recognisable pattern – the patient presents with symptoms and features that lead the physician to give a diagnosis of Crohn's disease. There is often pain; other symptoms include weight-loss (with or without anorexia), and a disturbed bowel habit (particularly diarrhoea, but this may not be helpful unless there are other features which suggest something other than a functional disorder).

The presence of blood and mucus signals large bowel disease. Abdominal distension, nausea and vomiting are quite common. Extra-intestinal manifestations are often helpful in diagnosis. One or more of the following, all of which can be associated with active Crohn's disease, should ensure that a diagnosis of Crohn's disease is considered:

- Pyoderma gangrenosum
- Erythema nodosum
- Conjunctivitis
- Episcleritis
- Iritis
- Perianal area problems, particularly fistulas and florid fleshy skin tags.

Abdominal pain, change of bowel habit and weight loss in a patient may indicate Crohn's disease. Biopsies of the skin tags often reveal characteristic granulomas. Again, as with ulcerative colitis, the coexistence of arthritis involving the large joints at a time when the bowel disease is active should make the physician consider inflammatory bowel disease.

It is unfortunate that Crohn's disease can occur anywhere within the gastrointestinal tract, from the lips to the anus, whereas in ulcerative colitis only the large bowel is affected. It is here that barium enema can be of value as it can show the characteristic changes of Crohn's disease in the colon. The radiological changes that can be seen are superficial and deep ulceration, oedematous and thickened mucosa, skip lesions, cobblestones, inflammatory polyps, and changes in the lumen such as narrowing, strictures, proximal dilatation and fistulas. Distinguishing between ulcerative colitis and Crohn's disease can be difficult. Pain is often a feature of Crohn's disease but not of ulcerative colitis. Ulceration of the bowel in Crohn's disease is deep and fissuring, and characteristically 'rose thorn' in type, whereas ulcerative colitis tends to be associated with more superficial ulceration. The presence of skin tags and perianal fistulas and strictures are also features that point towards Crohn's disease.

History and aetiology

The history of Crohn's disease has proved more elusive than the history of ulcerative colitis. German literature at the turn of the 19th century was full of references to obscure, non-specific granulomas but the condition did not become a clinical entity until 1932. In that year Burrill Bernard Crohn (born 1884) and his colleagues in New York described a disease they called 'regional ileitis'. The disease did not take kindly to being unmasked and the name 'regional ileitis' was shown to be a sad misconception. It ultimately proved that it could appear anywhere along the gastrointestinal tract from the mouth to the anus. At the present time we see Crohn's disease roughly as commonly in the large bowel as in the small bowel.

Once the disease is established, gastrointestinal physicians found that it was very difficult to treat, responding little, if at all, to medical measures, and surgery came quickly to the scene. The earliest note of ulcerative colitis was made by Giovani Batista Morgagni (1682–1771) when he saw a young man whose bowels were described as being afflicted with ulcers. In 1859 Samuel Wilkes of Guy's Hospital gave a recognisable description of ulcerative colitis. In 1891 Arthur William Mayo-Robson saw a woman of 37 whose colitis and proctitis with ulceration was only getting worse on medical treatment, and he resolved to cure the condition. He embarked on surgery for this woman and brought out the sigmoid colon to the surface and 4 days later opened the bowel. He then decided that a course of irrigation of water and boracic acid solution would help. He closed the artificial anus, and after an unspecified time, the patient reported back fit and well.

The aetiology of Crohn's disease remains unknown. There have been many suggestions such as bacteria, diet, environment and immunological abnormality. Since 1993, research linking the measles vaccine to Crohn's disease has threatened to jeopardise the efforts of the community health teams to fulfil the Department of Health's plans to eliminate the measles virus. The first published evidence, from the Royal Free Hospital's Inflammatory Bowel Study Group, appeared in 1994. The group used virus morphology to identify persistent measles virus in the intestinal cells of patients with Crohn's disease. At present, the published evidence suggesting such an association appears to be unconvincing and the Department of Health maintains its stance that the measles vaccine is safe (Kmietowicz 1997). Crohn's disease does not discriminate and it can affect anybody – young, old, man or woman.

Occasionally with the disease, abscesses, known as fistulas, can break through to the skin, allowing pus to escape. The illness will start with vague symptoms: tiredness, listlessness, lethargy, weight loss and diarrhoea. Often there will be mucus and blood. Some people have abdominal pain, skin tags and other symptoms of Crohn's as previously discussed.

Investigations

Investigations to aid diagnosis include the following:

- Small bowel enema: an X-ray where barium is passed into the small bowel. This will help to identify narrowings or strictures.
- Large bowel enema: a radiological diagnostic test where barium is introduced via the back passage to outline the large bowel, the colon. This will help to identify stricture and areas of inflammation (often at the ileocaecal junction).
- Colonoscopy

- Disease activity can be assessed by blood tests and radioactive isotope studies of the bowel.

Treatment

Initial treatment may take the form of medicine and diet. Surgery is often done as a last attempt to cure or keep the disease under control.

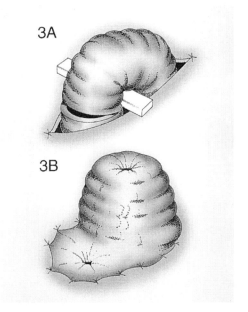

3A

3B

Figure 6.1 Loop ileostomy construction

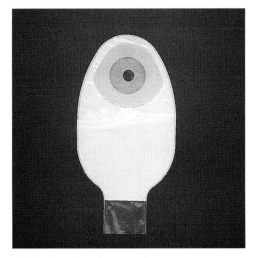

Figure 6.2 One-piece ileostomy bag

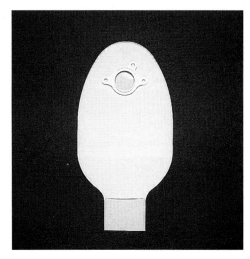

Figure 6.3 Two-piece ileostomy bag

Drugs

Various medications can be used, including steroids such as hydrocortisone, prednisone and prednisolone, all of which reduce inflammation. They can be taken as an injection in severe stages, or as infusions and tablets, taken normally when the patient is at home or in the form of suppositories or enemas into the rectum. Steroids are used to treat flare-ups of the disease but they do not stop the disease. Their use must be carefully controlled and they should never be stopped abruptly. Steroid dosages should always be tailed off gradually under the supervision of a medical practitioner and it is essential that patients carry a card stating that they are on steroids and the dose which they are currently taking in case of accident. It is known that steroids used over long periods in high doses can cause unwanted side-effects. These include an increase in weight, hair growth, Cushingnoid appearance (moon face), high blood pressure and reduction in bone density.

Other drugs used in Crohn's disease include sulphasalazine. The use of this medicine in Crohn's disease is less clear than in ulcerative colitis but it is thought that in some cases sulphasalazine may reduce the frequency of exacerbations of the disease. It has to be taken continuously, even if the disease appears not to be in its active stage.

Azathioprine acts in a similar way to steroids. It suppresses the immune system and reduces inflammation. It does not have the same side-effects as steroids but can lower the white blood cells which normally help to combat infection, and so can make the patient more susceptible to infections and diseases.

Metronidazole (Flagyl®) is an antibiotic which is often used in abdominal and gut surgery and to treat infections associated with bowel diseases. It can be used in short courses to treat abscesses around the anus. 6-mercaptopurine and cyclosporin are both used to suppress inflammation.

Diet

There is much interest in diet in the treatment of Crohn's disease. Many people will omit all dairy products from their diet and feel that this helps their disease process. Liquid diets which have little or no fibre are often used to rest the bowel. They can be given as enteral feeds when the patient is ill in hospital, but can also be taken as oral feeds at home. Liquid diets can be very effective in controlling exacerbations of Crohn's disease but compliance can be low as they taste unpleasant. Even elemental diets can be unpleasant and compliance again is difficult with patients at home and even in hospital.

Some Crohn's patients remove everything from their diet and bring back foods one by one, perhaps starting with something like chicken and mashed potato, and gradually adding other foods to see how their disease is affected.

Crohn's disease will often respond to medical treatment but for some patients, as with ulcerative colitis, surgery will be necessary. The effects of surgery and the type of surgery for both ulcerative colitis and Crohn's disease are discussed below.

SURGERY

The surgical management of ulcerative colitis

Ulcerative colitis affects more than 80 000 people in Britain and about 5000 people develop the disease each year (Stafford Miller 1993). It is more common among whites than blacks and the prevalence in Jewish people is 3 to 5 times that in non Jews (Kelly 1992). It affects men and women equally (Jones & Irving 1993) and most commonly occurs in the age range 20–40 years. In the most familial pattern, two or more children of a first-degree relative are affected (Kelly 1992). The disease is also reported to be more common in identical twins than in single births (Phillips 1995).

Of the many patients who suffer attacks of ulcerative colitis throughout their lifetime, only about 20–30% will undergo surgery to remove the diseased large colon. For many years the indications for surgery for ulcerative colitis have remained unchanged. They are: fulminating colitis with the risk of perforation or bleeding, malignant change, dysplasia, toxic dilatation of the colon, and failed medical treatment in patients with chronic disease.

Surgical options (see also Figs 6.1, 6.2, 6.3, and Plates 1 and 2)

Patients who are considering surgery may find an ileostomy unacceptable. They may have heard about it from others who have had the disease, or through associations such as the National Association of Colitis and Crohn's Disease or the Ileostomy Association. An ileostomy may nevertheless be required when the disease can no longer be adequately treated by other means.

Until the 1980s the normal course of action for the patient requiring surgery for management of ulcerative colitis resulting in an ileostomy was a proctocolectomy with ileostomy. The ileostomy was redesigned in 1952 by Brian Brooke and is now known as the Brooke ileostomy. Proctocolectomy with a Brooke ileostomy is considered to be the 'gold standard'. Even though this operation is curative and postoperative rehabilitation is straightforward, with the patient going back to work soon after surgery and returning to a normal life with a good quality of life, the thought of having a stoma is too much for some patients. For them the psychological and social price outweighs the advantages being offered.

One of the early alternatives to having a

proctocolectomy and ileostomy, resulting in a stoma, was to carry out a procedure of colectomy and ileorectal anastomosis. However, because in this procedure the rectum and anus are left in situ, a draw back is the risk of the malignancy returning to the rectum. An alternative to this is the Kock continent ileostomy (see Fig. 6.5), which provides a flush stoma underneath the skin. However, with this type of ileostomy the valve can become blocked with food and faecal output, leading to obstruction. Although the Kock reservoir (Kock 1969) offers the advantages of a classical proctocolectomy with a continent stoma, the patient does have to intubate the reservoir for emptying. There is a high incidence of valve failure as patients do come back with obstruction.

In 1978 Parks and Nicholls described a procto-colectomy without ileostomy for ulcerative colitis (Parks & Nicholls 1978) to which they added a reservoir by fashioning a pelvic pouch out of the terminal ileum. This became known as the Parks pouch (now generally known as the ileal–anal reservoir). The advantage of this reservoir is that the patient does not have an ileostomy and defecates through the normal back passage. Also the mucosa is stripped away from the rectum, so decreasing the risk of any malignancy returning.

Problems with proctocolectomy and ileostomy are that the perineal wound can take a long time to heal – often a year or even longer – and if the operation is undertaken by inexperienced hands there can be sexual dysfunction resulting from injury to the pelvic nerves.

Before any of these operations take place time is spent by the surgeon and the stoma care nurse in counselling the patient and the family on the type of operation chosen by the patient. The stoma care nurse will also have given the patient information about types of operation and discuss with the patient the type of operation which would be most suitable.

Panproctocolectomy (see Fig. 6.8, below) in-volves removal of the whole of the large bowel, including the rectum. The terminal end of the small bowel is brought onto the abdominal surface in the right iliac fossa as an ileostomy. This is known as an end ileostomy. About 6–7 cm of the small bowel is brought out onto the abdominal surface and inverted back and sewn to the abdominal wall. This is known as a Brooke ileostomy. This shortened spout (3–4 cm) is necessary to keep the extremely irritant effluent from the small bowel away from the abdominal skin. The spout of the ileostomy allows the effluent to go into the appliance. Removal of the rectum and anus eliminates the risk of bowel cancer, and the operation is a complete cure for ulcerative colitis.

With a continent ileostomy or Kock pouch (see Fig. 6.5, below) the internal reservoir is constructed from terminal ileum with an outlet valve to the body surface. The ileostomy reservoir or Kock pouch is managed by the patient, who intubates the pouch with a catheter and allows the effluent to run out into a jug or into the toilet. This operation is technically demanding and results are not always satisfactory (Coloplast 1995).

If an ileorectal anastomosis is performed this also side-steps the stoma and an ileostomy is not needed. It was once a popular alternative with patients, since the rectum is spared, but again, there is great danger of the recurrence in the rectum of malignant disease which may remain undiagnosed for a long period. Since the intro-duction of the Parks pouch, or ileal–anal reservoir, the operation is not now often performed, although sometimes it can be indicated for the older patient as it enables there to be relative rectal sparing. In cases of fulminating colitis and emergency surgery the operation of choice is now colectomy with terminal ileostomy and preservation of the rectal stump. This gives the patient the chance to recover and decide which procedure should be next. When a patient is admitted for emergency surgery there is no time for counselling or discussion of the advantages and disadvantages of the various types of ileostomy procedure. Preserving the rectal stump allows time for the patient to be counselled later and to make an informed decision on whether they want to undertake an ileal–anal reservoir or keep the ileostomy.

Colectomy with ileostomy and preservation of the rectal stump has a mortality of less than 5%. Using this as an emergency procedure allows the therapeutic options of ileorectal anastomosis (which is rarer these days), ileoanal reservoir or proctectomy to be undertaken at a later date.

A temporary loop ileostomy allows the whole colon to be rested without removing the large bowel. Refinements in surgical procedure in the last few years, together with the advent of far superior appliances, are leading to an increase in its popularity. Loop ileostomy is used to protect ileorectal and ileoanal anastomosis. It can be used as a second part of surgery covering an ileoanal reservoir, or following operations for the colon, diverticular disease or acute Crohn's disease of the rectum and anus. It then allows healing of the distal excision and lesions, especially fistulas.

In patients who require the formation of a stoma from the large bowel (the colon), loop ileostomy is preferable because it is easy to site well and in a way which facilitates good management, the effluent is relatively inoffensive and more predictable, and the stoma itself is less bulky. In some centres in the UK loop ileostomy is the first choice for temporary stoma. To make a loop ileostomy, a loop of ileum is brought through to the surface of the abdominal wall and supported on a plastic rod. After the ileum has been cut round two-thirds of its circumference on one side of the loop, a spout can be formed from the longer arm of the loop (Coloplast 1995).

Surgery for Crohn's disease

Crohn's disease often responds to medication but sometimes, due to strictures or severe inflammation, it may be necessary for a piece of the affected bowel to be removed. Like ulcerative colitis, Crohn's disease can present as an emergency for surgery and the indications for urgent surgery in both diseases are identical. But in addition, in Crohn's disease, there may be perforation or abscess formation or fistula formation. If there is abscess formation this may require drainage and sometimes defunctioning of the bowel with a stoma can be considered.

The indications for elective surgery in Crohn's disease are the same as for ulcerative colitis. Although there is a cancer risk it is considerably

lower in Crohn's disease. Permanent stoma will be necessary when removal of the anal sphincter mechanism is undertaken. Indications for proctectomy include severe rectal disease, severe anal disease or both.

The incidence of anal Crohn's disease is greater the more distal the intestinal involvement; when it is confined to the small intestine the incidence is 10–15% compared with 50–80% when there is rectal involvement (Hellers et al 1980).

Proctocolectomy is the operation of choice when anal–rectal disease is combined with colonic involvement. In this situation the reoperative rate for recurrence is low at 10–30% at 5 years. It is noted that in 50% of patients with large bowel Crohn's disease there is rectal sparing. When a colectomy with ileal–rectal anastomosis is suitable the recurrence rate requiring further surgery is high at around 50% at 5 years (Allen et al 1977). Recurrence when it occurs is usually in the terminal ileum up to the anastomosis site. Sometimes it is possible to resect the anastomosis site and re-anastomose healthy small intestine to the rectum.

Some patients who have aggressive Crohn's disease or who require several resections of small bowel and have had a proctocolectomy may only be left with a small intestinal stoma of the upper ileum or jejunum. These patients are at risk of water and electrolyte imbalances and nutritional deficiency due to the fact that they are unable to absorb enough protein, calories and vitamins, especially vitamin B_{12}. They tend to fall into the category of high output ileostomies.

Because the output from an ileostomy is semi-solid on a good day and can be like very fluid porridge on a bad day and is known as effluent, there is potential danger to the skin if leakage occurs. Unpleasant odours are not usually a serious problem for ileostomists. (Odour and appliances are considered in Ch. 9).

Ileostomy action cannot be controlled – and no new ileostomy patient should be misled on this point – but it can be helped. Ileostomy output is generally active within half an hour to 1 hour after the main meal and less active at other times. The amount of effluent cannot be curtailed by taking less food and drink and it is very important that ileostomists take in a high intake of fluid to stabilise their water balance. Once the large colon has been removed and an ileostomy or ileoanal reservoir is in place, the body is less efficient at retaining salt and water, though the ability to digest food is normal. It is particularly important for patients to drink plenty of fluid after their ileostomy operation because at first the output of the stoma contains more liquid, but over a period of time the stools should become less fluid as the small intestine reabsorbs some of the fluid into the body.

The results of surgery for those with ulcerative colitis or for those needing an ileostomy or colostomy after Crohn's disease are greatly improved, and most patients find that they feel much better and have a good recovery. Modern surgery offers a number of options for those who have to follow this path but good counselling from a stoma care nurse and the consultant allow an informed choice to be made. Stoma surgery also gives a good quality of life and patients undergoing ileostomy for ulcerative colitis can expect a normal lifespan. Two illustrative case studies follow.

Case study: Proctocolectomy with ileostomy: Alma

I first met Alma 10 years after her first operation for ulcerative colitis. She had met the surgeon when surgery was first contemplated and had been offered an ileostomy to cure her, but she had refused. She had also been seen by a nurse who had shown her a bag which she found quite unacceptable to her personal body image and style. Because Alma did not want to have an ileostomy at that stage (or indeed at any time), ileorectal anastomosis was undertaken and over the next 10 years, between the ages of 40 and 50, there had been many operations to try to relieve the stricture until, ultimately, the surgeon said he could do no more and ileostomy would have to be undertaken.

When I met Alma she was a very upset lady. In fact, when we sat down to talk, she said that because of the ileorectal anastomosis and her lack of control over it during the last 10 years she had rarely been out. Her children had had children and she was unable to enjoy them. Also, she could tell me with clarity every public toilet within a 25-mile radius of her house. Any time she went out she would have 10, 15, or 20 minutes until she had to go to the toilet again. She would be wearing pads and she would have soiled underwear. She was aware that she smelled and this caused her quality of life to be extremely poor and gradually led to her becoming more and more reclusive and reluctant to leave her house. She had a very supportive relationship with her husband who unfortunately did not seem to be able to get her to get more out of life.

The final blow came when she attended the outpatient follow-up clinic and the surgeon said that this time he could not undertake any more stretching of the stricture from the ileorectal anastomosis – further surgery would have to take place resulting in an ileostomy. It was at this stage that I was introduced to her and discussed with her the outcomes of ileostomy and her fears and problems. I took with me one of the modern bags that were on the market at that time and which had proved successful for most of my patients. When I showed her the bag I was unprepared for the result – she just laughed at me and she said I was pulling her leg and being rather silly and

that this was not a bag. Apparently she had previously been shown a very old-fashioned bag that was extremely long (over 12 in) and had said that there was no way she could wear that under her clothes. This was the main reason why she had not contemplated having an ileostomy. When I showed her this new bag on the market and how low profile it was, how thin, how light, she actually said 'Can I have the operation tomorrow?' Obviously we had to plan for this but she was relieved to see that improvements in appliances had taken place.

Alma had her operation and used her bag. She was a very big lady and it took some time for her to get used to her body shape because of the fat folds, although we had sited the ileostomy in the most acceptable place for her to manage for the rest of her life. I followed up Alma at home for the first 2 months or so and we had long chats. She was a happy, bouncy, bubbly lady then; life had totally changed for her. Although she was still feeling weak after the operation she was doing more around the house, she was going out more in the car with her husband, and she was beginning to get back to going shopping, which was her delight. Her other major delight, unfortunately, was chocolate and her weight was also increasing because of her improved health. We did talk about this and tried to get Alma to eat sensibly and healthily by cutting out a good deal of the chocolate and the cakes but she found this difficult. Alma now manages her ileostomy extremely well, her output is well controlled, and more recently, in the yearly follow-ups that there have been for the last 2–3 years, she has told us all about her trips out and her holidays, things that she never had before or could ever discuss.

Alma shows that correct management, correct counselling and help, psychological and psychosocial support, helps patients to manage and to have a better quality of life. The stoma therapist can help patients to explore their fears within their lifestyle and can spend time with the patient and the family, allowing adaptation to take place and be successful even if a permanent ileostomy with an appliance is the outcome.

Case study: Crohn's disease: John

John was referred to the surgeons from the gastrointestinal physicians, and had been diagnosed as having Crohn's disease. He was not responding now to medication and was becoming unwell. He had weight loss, loss of appetite and lethargy, and had been medically discharged from his job at the very early age of 29. John had a wife and two young children and was feeling very down about his quality of life, and his possible job prospects; he was quite upset at the thought that he might not be able to go back to work and earn an income to support his young family, although his wife was working.

The surgeons considered that an operation would be needed and an ileostomy would be the best outcome for John. It was discussed with John and it was decided that a panproctocolectomy with permanent end ileostomy would be the route taken. A lot of time was spent with John and his wife discussing the operation and the outcomes and his ultimate recovery. The discussions covered such topics as what types of jobs John could apply for after his recovery, his sexual competency after the operation and whether there would be any problems, and his whole lifestyle.

John underwent his surgery and made an uneventful recovery. Although there were some very good low-profile one-piece ileostomy bags on the market, John ultimately opted for a two-piece drainable appliance, which he thought would be easier and would fit in better with his lifestyle.

The perineal area took a while to get better and to dry up, and the wound had some minor discharge from one part for longer than would be expected. John was seen in outpatients 6 or 8 weeks later and felt considerably better, although he was still recovering and in his rehabilitation period. He was beginning to think about work and what he could do, and about whether there would be any restrictions because of his ileostomy. At his second outpatient appointment at 3 months John was found to have a healed perineal area, a healed wound and an ileostomy that was working well. He was feeling much better in himself and was beginning to make applications for further jobs. At 6 months John referred himself back to the stoma clinic complaining of perineal leaking, a greeny, mucky discharge through a very small pinhole type sinus in the perineal area. This was being treated with antibiotics from the doctor but had now been going on for a month. The discharge was enough to make a mark and stain his clothes and was offensive in odour. Swabs were taken and a further course of antibiotics started. It was felt necessary to let the district nurses know so that the perineal area could be packed in an effort to cure this sinus. The sinus gradually appeared to be healing, drainage stopped, antibiotics were finished and John carried on with his life. Fourteen months later John again self-referred to the stoma clinic with perineal leakage, offensive odour, green discharge. Again, antibiotics had been started by the GP. John was also finding he had a lot of perineal pain, especially after sexual intercourse. A sinogram was undertaken but was found to be a dead end. There did not seem to be any obvious reason why he was having this continual drainage which suddenly broke down and started and then healed. It was decided to take him back into hospital and to do a small resection of the perineal area to clean out any sutures which were annoying him (or perhaps he had an allergy to the internal sutures) and to re-sew the small part of the perineal area. This was done and John went home feeling much happier and more comfortable within the perineal area.

John returned to the stoma clinic as a self-referral $2\frac{1}{2}$ years after the perineal resection saying that the same thing was happening again. He was having perineal pain, pain after intercourse, there was a discharge build up, and a foul, offensive odour. The GP had again started antibiotics and the district nurse had been called to irrigate and pack the wound. Again a small sinus was found and a sinogram showed a dead end sinus. Again it was considered whether to take him back to theatre to do a minor procedure and a clearing out. This continual leakage was becoming too much for John. He had found himself another job but the pain and discharge were interfering with his lifestyle and his job. It was therefore decided to admit him into day-care and clean out the perineal area, again with a small resection, and see what the outcome was. This was ultimately done and John went home. For over a year now John has had a less painful perineal area and no discharge and no need for continual antibiotics.

It does appear that in Crohn's disease this sort of thing can happen. The perineal area or the wound can break down, and this can go on for quite a long time and be quite debilitating. Patients with Crohn's disease who have a complete recovery with no subsequent problems like this are the luckier ones but careful management and help and not allowing the problem to continue may have helped to resolve the problem in John's case although it took in excess of $3\frac{1}{2}$ years. John has now settled down into a new job and his family are beginning to grow up and he and his wife are enjoying their quality of life together. Even though he has a permanent end ileostomy he feels this is far more satisfactory than being ill with Crohn's disease.

Surgical procedures (Figs 6.4–6.6) (see also Figs 6.7–6.11, below)

In 1978 Parks & Nicholls described a surgical procedure to avoid a permanent ileostomy. This has become one of the major developments in surgery for patients with inflammatory bowel disease, very specifically either ulcerative colitis or patients who may suffer familial polyposis. For the moment this type of procedure is not suitable for patients who have the inflammatory bowel disease known as Crohn's disease.

Restorative proctocolectomy was pioneered at St Mark's Hospital by Sir Alan Parks and John Nicholls and initially it was known as a Parks pouch. Although this sort of procedure offers a certain group of patients the opportunity to avoid a permanent ileostomy, as with all new procedures it has to be recognised that there are significant complications both physically and psychologically. Restorative proctocolectomy is also known under various terms, most commonly an ileal–anal pouch (Parks, Nicholls & Belliveaus 1980). (See Figs 6.4–6.6.)

Procedures can differ and the surgical technique used in the construction of the final configuration of the pouch is often given an alphabetical attachment such as the 'J' pouch, 'S' pouch, or 'W' pouch. The original Parks pouch, first described by Sir Alan Parks, was constructed using three loops of ileum of up to 50 cm and was formed into an 'S' shape. More recently other pouch shapes have emerged. The 'W' shaped pouch was described by Nicholls & Loboski in 1987. This provides a pouch that is able to hold the largest volume. The pouch incorporates 60 cm of terminal ileum, and the procedure involves resection of the colon and proximal rectum with stripping of the mucosal surface of the distal rectum and construction of the ileal pouch with ileal–anal anastomosis. Often the newly formed pouch is protected by a temporary loop ileostomy which can be closed at a later stage when the extensive suture lines are settled within the pouch surgery.

When deciding whether a particular patient is suitable for this procedure it is important to define the aims of such surgery and important that the patient fully understands. This will ensure that the final outcome will be the best for the patient. Good recovery from the surgery depends greatly on thorough preoperative counselling and understanding by the patient and his immediate carers of what the operation will entail and of the recovery procedure, and understanding that recovery is not instant.

Although an ileostomy could be avoided by an ileal–anal anastomosis or an ileal–rectal anastomosis, these may result in frequent bowel output and may not be satisfactory for the patient. Having a restorative proctocolectomy that makes a reservoir helps the patient to have less frequent bowel motions and also to avoid having a stoma and bag. Patients undergoing the procedure must be fit at the time of surgery from the anaesthetist and surgeon's point of view. Although many patients are still taking steroids at the time of surgery, dosages should be as low as possible. It has been found that the patient who is on 10 mg or less to no steroids may well fare better after surgery, with good healing. The advantage of having restorative proctocolectomy, especially for the patient with ulcerative colitis, is that all drugs can cease after surgery. If the patient has been on a larger amount of steroids these will be tailed off over the next few weeks.

Age does not seem to be a determinant against having restorative surgery to avoid ileostomy. Patients in the older age bracket (65 years of age or over) or exceptionally young must be carefully considered. Although the procedure for restorative proctocolectomy is now becoming a fairly normal option for patients in most district general hospitals where there is a surgeon who is happy to undertake it, patients in the very young age group or in the older age group may need to be referred elsewhere. Patients below the age of 16 should perhaps be referred to a paediatric centre with surgeons who are aware of all the problems with paediatric colorectal surgery.

A major requirement for a good outcome from this type of surgery is good anal sphincter function. It is known that muscles deteriorate with ageing, and so it can also be expected that the anal sphincter will deteriorate with ageing. This may lead to an increased problem after restorative proctocolectomy in people aged over 55–60. This procedure should therefore be considered very carefully, but not necessarily disregarded.

Preoperative preparation

It is extremely important that the patient and the patient's carers, spouse, partners, and anyone else involved in their well-being understand what the outcomes are likely to be. Patients who have had good preoperative counselling and time spent with them and their families in going

The suppositories need to be held in place, either by a piece of gauze over the colostomy or by the patient holding a hand over the appliance for about 20 minutes, to allow time for the suppositories to melt.

If a colonoscopy or contrast study is to be performed, stringent bowel cleansing is needed.

If the patient is to undergo colonic surgery the bowel must be totally free of faecal matter as faecal contamination of the wound or peritoneal cavity can cause sepsis and wound complications such as infection and dehiscence. In severe circumstances, multi organ failure may occur.

The patient is usually admitted 2 days before surgery so that bowel preparation can begin and the patient is advised to have a low residue diet, followed by a day of clear fluids to help the cleansing of the bowel. The day before surgery the patient is given a laxative which causes

diarrhoea. For the elderly patient this is extremely distressing, as often they cannot control the urgency. If they are not able to walk easily or see well, there may be difficulty for them in getting to the toilet. This should be assessed before giving the bowel preparation and if possible the patient given an en suite room prior to surgery. If this is not possible, a commode should be available at the bedside.

Some elderly patients may be undernourished before surgery and the giving of a laxative with the resulting diarrhoea can severely upset their electrolytes. Patients should be closely supervised when taking a bowel preparation to ensure that they finish all the required liquid and do not dispose of it down the sink. Poor preparation of the colon may result in the unexpected need for a stoma if an expected anastomosis cannot be undertaken due to faecal contamination.

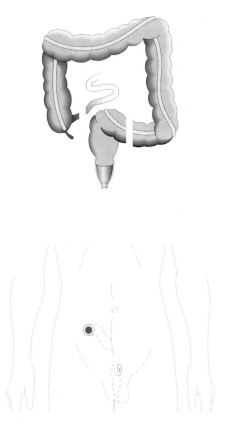

Figure 6.9 Total colectomy, rectal stump retained

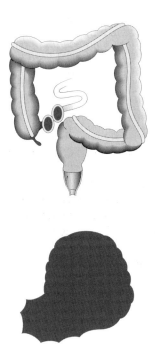

Figure 6.10 Loop ileostomy

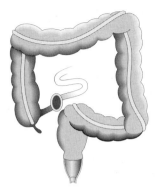

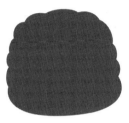

Figure 6.11   End ileostomy

Patients whose bowels are obstructed cannot have a laxative for bowel cleansing, but a distal colon washout may be given. Patients who have a perforated bowel can only be starved before surgery. Problems for patients can arise when bowel cleansing and starvation take place and the procedure or surgery is cancelled. If this happens frequently the patient who is elderly and frail may become quite ill.

Bowel preparation is not pleasant for the patient and can be embarrassing and upsetting if the patient is unable to control the output. Many elderly patients have never been incontinent in their lives and have never dirtied their bed, and they can be mortified when this happens. They must be given reassurance to help their anxiety levels and must be encouraged to drink plenty of water while taking the bowel preparation to avoid dehydration.

Box 6.4   Patient preparation for bowel procedures

Small bowel
Procedure
Contrast studies and barium swallow with intermittent films as contrast passes through small bowel
Purpose
Diagnosis of benign or malignant disease, stenosis, fistulae or anastomotic leaks
Preparation
Low residue diet, enema or laxative beforehand
Rationale
To allow unhindered transit of barium through the ileum and to clear the colon of any faeces that may obscure loops of small bowel filled with contrast
Colon
Procedure
Colonoscopy
Purpose
Screening for familial polyposis, ulcerative colitis, Crohn's disease, malignant disease
Preparation
Purgative one day beforehand, possible enema or washout
Rationale
To clean colon, as faecal matter will obscure view and diagnosis
Colon and rectum
Procedure
Contrast studies
Purpose
To diagnose any of the above conditions
Preparation
Clear fluids for 24 hours and oral purgatives
Rationale
To clear loaded faecal matter
Sigmoid colon
Procedure
Flexible sigmoidoscopy and rigid sigmoidoscopy
Purpose
As for colonoscopy
Preparation
Enema before procedure for flexible sigmoidoscopy. None for rigid unless the rectum is full of faeces
Rationale
Clear distal colon, sigmoid colon and rectum
Rectum
Procedure
Proctoscopy
Purpose
Investigate rectal bleeding, lesions, haemorrhoids, anal fissures, infective lesions
Preparation
As above
Abdomen
Procedure
Plain abdominal X-ray
Purpose
Diagnose bowel perforation or obstruction
Preparation
None. Will have been starved as will probably be an emergency admission
Rationale
First test to see the reason for acute abdominal pain

7

Urinary diversions

UROSTOMY

Urostomy is the general term given to the diversion of the urinary tract resulting in a stoma which is invariably permanent (see Fig. 7.1). A urinary diversion known as an ileal conduit, described by Bricker in 1950, was formerly the gold standard and the most popular form of urinary diversion.

The common reasons for a urinary diversion are:

- Carcinoma of the bladder or urethra
- Neuropathic bladder due to spinal column disorders
- Urinary incontinence (this may arise from trauma in childbirth or interstitial cystitis).

When carcinoma of the bladder is diagnosed the tumours are staged so that the degree of spread can be ascertained. The staging of tumours is as follows:

T1s In situ carcinoma
TA Papillary – no invasion of basement membrane
T1   Invasion of lamina propria
T2   Invasion of superficial muscle
T3a Invasion of deep muscle
T3b Invasion of perivesical fat
T4   Invasion of adjacent organ or bone.

It is estimated that there are about 2000 new urostomies raised each year in the UK, despite the fact that there have been major advances in reconstructive surgery in the last 10 years. For many patients who require a urinary diversion, the urostomy is the operation of choice. A portion of ileum about 30 cm long is isolated with its mesentery vessels from an area close to the ileocaecal junction. This is to ensure that the maximum amount of ileum remains to allow the continued function of bile salt and vitamin B_{12} absorption. The identified piece of ileum with its mesentery is mobilised and the distal end is attached to the peritoneum and the remaining ends of the bowel are anastomosed to restore the bowel continuity.

The ureters are implanted into the closed proximal end of the isolated segment after being resected from the bladder, often following the Wallace technique (1970). The distal end of the segment of bowel is brought on to the right side of the abdominal wall as a stoma with a spout as described by Brooke (1952) in the construction of the Brooke ileostomy. The stoma should arise on the right side of the abdominal wall through the rectus abdominis muscle to help alleviate the possible problem of peristomal hernia.

Preoperative care

Care given to patients prior to surgery for urinary diversion will help to allay their fears about the forthcoming operation and their recovery. As with all stoma operations, ideally counselling should start as soon as the patient is informed of the diagnosis and the need for the operation, in the outpatient department. However, the news given by the doctor is often as much as patients and relatives are able to absorb at this point. It is often better for stoma therapists to introduce themselves, leave a contact number, and explain to patients that it is better to see them in their own surroundings in a couple of days for a discussion about all the aspects of the forthcoming operation and the return to normal living. This gives both the patient and his or her family time to absorb the consultation with the doctor and to start to formulate the questions and worries that they have about the urinary diversion.

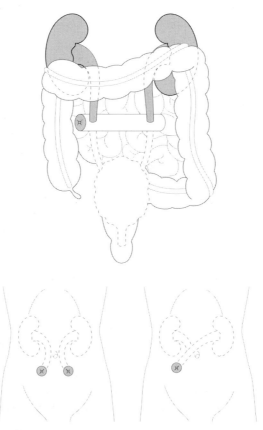

Figure 7.1 Common urostomy procedures

Other specific preoperative investigations will be undertaken before the operation for the formation of a urostomy. They are:

- Renal function tests: these determine glomerular filtration and creatinine clearance from the kidneys. If this is not adequate, surgery may not be able to go ahead.
- Intravenous urography: this outlines the renal and lower drainage system to show structural or possible drainage problems.
- CT (computerised tomography) scan: this determines the extent of the disease and the involvement of any other structures.

The patient will be admitted 2 days before surgery for bowel preparation. It is common practice in most hospitals today to see the patient a week before this to check their preoperative status at a preoperative clinic. This allows a reduction in the length of time that patients are admitted to hospital before surgery. In the 2 days before surgery, bowel preparation is given in the form of sodium picosulphate (or whatever preparation is the urologist's preference). Bowel preparation is helped if the patient has been on clear fluids for 48 hours before hospital admission. Often intravenous fluid is needed whilst the patient is undergoing bowel cleansing and prior to surgery, to maintain hydration.

Postoperative care

Although nursing care is the same as after any major abdominal surgery, there are some specifics that are imperative to the postoperative care of the urostomy patient and there may be stomal complications in the early days after surgery.

One of the main differences in a urinary stoma compared with faecal stomas is the presence of urinary stents. These are fine-bore catheters (quite often paediatric naso-gastric tubes) that are inserted via the new stoma up into the anastomosis and just beyond into each ureter to maintain the patency and protect the suturing until primary healing is completed. Stents are usually left in situ for 7–10 days and removed just before the patient is discharged home. Changing the appliance can prove difficult for the patient whilst the stents

are in situ and help and guidance from the nurse will be needed. Occasionally the urologist may require the stents to be left in longer than 10 days, especially if the patient has had prior radiotherapy to the bladder. The patency of the stents should be checked regularly in the immediate postoperative period and, if necessary, they should be flushed through with saline to prevent any mucous blockage. When the urostomy appliance is put on, the stents should be passed through the non-return valve of the pouch to enable the drained urine to pass into the pouch beyond the non-return valve and not come into contact with the newly formed stoma and the adhesive of the pouch. When the stents are removed the patient is often fearful that it will be painful. Full explanation of the procedure and reassurance should be given. Usually pulling of the stents with a little gentle traction is enough to release them and they will come away. Sometimes this may be difficult and the patient becomes anxious, but repeating the procedure on a daily basis will often enable the stents to come out. Quite often one stent or the other falls out before the 7–10 days.

Urostomy appliances (see Figs 7.2 and 7.3 below, and Plates 3–5)

Patients who are confident in the care of their urostomy may want choose the appliance from the urostomy range that suits them best, and this may be either a one-piece or a two-piece appliance. However, if the urostomy is new, the patient will often be guided by the nurse or stoma care specialist as to which appliance will be best in the early days and months. The majority of urostomy patients in the UK wear a light-weight, disposable plastic appliance, attached with an adhesive, in the form of a one-piece or two-piece appliance. Urostomy bags have a non-return valve inside to prevent backflow of urine onto the stoma and peristomal skin. The nurse or stoma therapist will help the patient with the correct choice of appliance by taking into account the patient's manual dexterity, visual ability, skin contours and patient choice of appliance with guidance from the nurse or stoma therapist (Ostomy Patients' Charter, see Appendix).

The urostomy pouch can be clear or opaque, a one-piece or two-piece system, both with a hydrocolloid adhesive backing. Patients with an active lifestyle may find the two-piece system offers distinct advantages in allowing the pouches to be changed quickly and easily, but without removing the adhesive each time. One of the earliest two-piece systems was developed by Convatec in 1978, and, as with all appliances, the two-piece system has been improved in recent years. Many of the other ostomy manufacturers saw the advantage of a two-piece system and now there are several two-piece systems for the patient to choose from. Most urostomy pouches come in two sizes, small and standard, and both have non-return valves. All urostomy bags will have a secure tap on the end and this will be either a fold-up tap or a swivel tap. The swivel tap turns until a coloured mark is seen to indicate that the tap is open ready for drainage. The advantage of this type of tap is that the coloured point has an indentation as well which makes it a suitable appliance for the urostomy patient who is blind or has only partial sight. The shorter urostomy pouches are suitable for people who are of shorter stature or smaller build, or for short-term wear during sporting activities.

It is important that the flange or one-piece bag is cut to the correct size of the urostomy so that it fits snugly around the stoma. In hospital, during postoperative recovery, the aperture in the flange or one-piece appliance is cut to size from a starter hole, but once the stoma has settled down – up to 1 month after surgery – a pre-cut flange or pre-cut one-piece appliance can be ordered. A flange should be at least 6 mm larger than the diameter of the stoma.

Some stomas can be difficult to manage because they are flush to the skin or in a skin fold, or even below the skin level. In situations such as these leaking may occur under and around the flange, causing a distressing management problem for the patient. Often a filler paste, available on prescription, will solve this problem. The paste is applied to the indentations and gullies near the stoma to even up the surface to enable the flange or one-piece appliance to adhere comfortably and securely. If paste does not solve the

leakage problem, a convex flange may help. Convexity works by pushing the area around the stoma inwards, making the stoma protrude. The extra pressure convexity applies improves the contact between the skin and the skin barrier to help prevent leakage. The controlled use of convexity in situations such as these can often prevent a patient returning to theatre for revision of the urostomy.

Convexity should only be used under medical or nursing supervision as inappropiate use may lead to a damaged stoma. For adult patients who have a urostomy there is the problem of night-time drainage. Because the pouch can only take a limited amount of urine, it needs to be emptied during the night, and patients can find this disturbing to their sleep pattern. To allow the continuity of the sleep pattern, companies making urostomy pouches also make a connecting night drainage system. The night drainage system is suitable for use with a one-piece or a two-piece appliance. The night drainage bag has a non-return valve to prevent the backflow of urine into the pouch and has long, flexible tubing allowing for movement in bed. It has holes to take a carrying handle or for attachment to floor-standing drainage stands, beds or wheelchairs. The bottom of the night drainage bag has a tap that is easy to open and close for drainage. Also available are night bags to attach to the pouch with a tap rather than a flip-end closure. The advantage of this is that it incorporates a swivel connection to allow greater freedom of movement. When patients use a pouch system that has a tap (as previously described), a leg bag may also be attached. This allows for an extra 500 ml capacity, which is especially useful for long journeys where there may not be the chance to empty the pouch in a toilet. This system is also useful for patients who are in wheelchairs. Occasionally patients feel very insecure when their urostomy pouch starts to fill and they find that the urostomy appears to be a lot heavier than an ileostomy or colostomy bag. A belt may give these patients added security and will help to support the weight of the bag. The belt can be attached to the belt lugs on either side of the urostomy bag, or a belt plate is available which passes over the appliance against the flange and the belt attaches to this. Many women wear an adapted pantie girdle or corset which also gives light-weight abdominal support.

Problem solving

Patients quite often experience problems once they are back in the community (although many of these are straightforward), and worry about any changes that they see. For example the urine may look cloudy and have strands of mucus in it. The patient assumes that infection is present and may contact his or her GP, who may prescribe antibiotics. The answer may be uncomplicated, and all that the patient is seeing is the mucus that is present in the piece of bowel that has been used for the diversion. Daily administration of ascorbic acid 100 mg (vitamin C) will clear the urine of excessive mucus and make the urine a golden colour (excess ascorbic acid in the body is excreted via the urinary system and a side-effect is to make the urine a golden colour). However, the GP must be consulted if the urine appears cloudy and has an offensive smell, accompanied by pain, raised temperature and chills, and in this case antibiotics may well be needed. It is also important that oral fluid level is kept high. Blood in the urine may occur for several reasons. The stoma may be caught by the flange (especially during changing). The stoma is particularly friable and can bleed with mis-handling. If the size of aperture of the flange is incorrect there may be friction between the stoma and the flange, resulting in stomal ulceration and bleeding. Infections may also give rise to blood in the urine.

Common causes of skin irritation around the stoma after urostomy include allergies to adhesives or the plastic of the urostomy pouch. Inflammation of the hair follicles may occur when the adhesives are removed for appliance change, especially in men. Regular, careful shaving of the area may help to prevent this. Constant leakage of urine from under the flange may result in irritated skin and help may be needed to rectify this situation. Referral back to the stoma care nurse may be necessary.

ALTERNATIVES TO UROSTOMY

For over a century urologists have been devising new techniques to side-step the operation that results in a urostomy. Continent urinary diversions are becoming increasingly available in many centres and one such alternative that would be suitable for some patients is the Mitrofanoff procedure (Leaver 1993). This new concept of a continent urinary diversion was first described by Paul Mitrofanoff, a French paediatric surgeon, in the 1980s. Since Mitrofanoff's first description of the pouch there have been two modifications (known as Mitrofanoff 2 and Mitrofanoff 3).

In the original pouch the appendix is utilised and becomes a catheterable port to release the urine. It is dissected on its mesentery and the caecal end brought to the abdominal surface as a stoma and the distal end cut off and channelled into the patient's bladder. As the bladder fills the ureters close naturally by the rising bladder pressure and the continent stoma also seals off. Intermittent catheterisation by the patient takes place as necessary. In this first type of pouch the patient's own bladder is preserved and used.

Mitrofanoff 2 involves a transuretero-ureterostomy and uses a piece of ureter as a catheterisable stoma. The bladder neck is closed and one ureter is anastomosed to the other. The distal end is bought out as a stoma.

Mitrofanoff 3 is suitable for patients who have had radical pelvic surgery or who may have a non-neuropathic bladder. A reservoir is made from bowel and the appendix is used as a non-return valve. The ileocaecal segment is opened along its border to make a large flattened expanse. This will provide a low pressure reservoir which the ureters are sewn into. The stoma can be sited anywhere on the abdominal wall (Randles 1992).

It cannot be emphasised enough that the patient must be given full, clear counselling if there is a choice of surgery between a urostomy or a reservoir, and decisions must not be made in a hurry. The patient should be seen with another member of his or her family so that the patient can discuss all the outcomes after counselling. Written information should be given on the appropriate types of surgery offered so that the patient can take them away to read. A contact number should be given to enable the patient to contact the stoma care nurse with any further questions before surgery.

Both internal reservoirs and urostomies have disadvantages and advantages. In the case of the reservoir these are as follows:

- The result is aesthetically more acceptable for body image as there is no appliance to wear
- There is no urine leakage
- Self-motivation is needed.
- It is a major complex operation
- Multiple scarring will occur
- Formation of stones in the reservoir
- Patient catheterisation is needed every 4–6 hours
- Long-term problems associated with this procedure are as yet unknown.

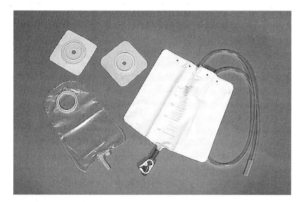

Figure 7.2 Urostomy appliances

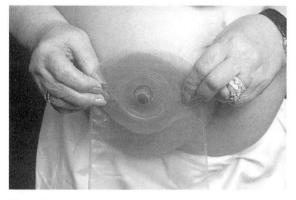

Figure 7.3 Urostomy bag

In the case of the urostomy they are:

- This is a well recognised procedure (Bricker procedure)
- Surgery is less extensive if the bladder is left in situ
- Caring for the appliance is a simple procedure
- The patient needs to wear a pouch at all times
- There may be difficulty in accepting the stoma
- There may be problems with body image
- There is a continual outflow of urine from the stoma.

Postoperative care of the reservoir patient differs from that of the urostomy patient, although normal observations after major abdominal surgery apply. As well as the normal observations the patient will have a catheter in the new channel and a suprapubic catheter, as well as drainage tubes. If the patient's ureter has been used as the channel (Mitrofanoff 2) there may be one or two ureteric stents in situ. The suprapubic and pouch catheters are flushed twice a day with 20 ml sterile saline or water for the first 3 days. Patients can take over the flushing of the catheters as soon as they are able, as they will have to continue this at home.

If ureteric stents are in place they are normally removed on day 10. A pouchogram is done after the 10th day to check the anastomosis and to confirm that there are no leaks in the pouch. If there is no dye leak, the suprapubic catheter is removed and the urine is drained via the pouch catheter in the stoma.

At home patients carry on with bladder washouts via the pouch catheter at least twice daily. After 4 weeks they are readmitted for the catheter to be clamped and fluid given so that they can experience the feeling of a distending bladder, a sensation which may be new to them. The clamp is removed after 2–4 hours, depending on the patient's ability to tolerate the new sensations. This procedure is repeated again to expand the pouch and to reach the expanded amount of 500 ml. Patients should be advised to empty the pouch every 4–6 hours and not allow the pouch to overfill as damage to the pouch may occur. After pouch stretching, the catheter is removed and the patient is taught to catheterise the pouch prior to discharge. On discharge patients are supplied with catheters and washout equipment and are referred to their local stoma care nurse. If there is no stoma care nurse available in their area, patients keep in touch with the hospital where the surgery was done. Because these operations are relatively new, GPs are generally inexperienced in the care of such patients and unable to give the appropriate care and advice.

Complications

Complications after this type of surgery depend on the extent of the surgery. Problems can occur in the pouch, the stoma or the continence mechanism. Experience now in this new surgery enables possible common complications to be anticipated in the postoperative period:

Incontinence

If the pouch becomes too full there may be overflow via the stoma. Reassessment of the way the pouch is being catheterised and encouraging the patient to drink more fluid may help. If pressure in the reservoir is not a problem, there may be a construction fault in the valve and surgery may be needed.

Stenosis of the stoma

This will cause difficulty in catheterising the pouch and a smaller catheter may be needed.

Acidosis

When urine is stored in an intestinal reservoir, metabolic changes may occur. Monitoring of electrolytes, magnesium, calcium and ammonium is important.

Stone formation

Stones occur through infection and mucus that is retained in the reservoir. The use of cranberry juice and reservoir washouts may help to prevent stone formation.

Reservoir rupture

This is due to over-extension of the reservoir and the loss of normal sensations.

Kidney damage

This may occur following repeated kidney infections, reflux, obstruction and urinary infection (Busuttil-Leaver 1994).

Patients are encouraged to have a high fluid intake (at least 3 litres per day) and, as previously described, the use of ascorbic acid and drinking 200 ml of cranberry juice per day, which acts as a bacteriostatic agent, help to keep the urine free from infection. Cranberry juice has been shown to inhibit bacterial adherence in *Escherichia coli* in vitro and in vivo, which suggests that there is prevention of adherence and colonisation of mucosal surfaces (Sobota 1984). There are several ways in which cranberry juice can be used in nursing practice and the clinical situations are:

- As a preventive measure against urinary tract infection
- As part of treatment for urinary tract infections
- To help prevent stone formation and growth
- To acidify the urine of patients who have urostomies and reservoirs
- To reduce mucus quantity and adherence (Busuttil-Leaver 1994).

CYSTOPLASTY

For some patients, enlargement of the bladder when part has been removed enables them to avoid a urostomy. This procedure is called a cystoplasty. For this the patient needs to learn self-catheterisation as there is a possibility that the bladder may not be able to be emptied properly, or at all. The patient must be made fully aware that, where a cytoplasty does not work, a urostomy may be the final answer.

A piece of detubularised bowel such as ileum or colon is used to increase the capacity of the bladder, and this known as an augmentation cystoplasty. The bladder can be removed nearly in total and a bladder refashioned using caecum,

---

Box 9.1 Factors to be considered when choosing an appliance

The person choosing the appliance, whether the stoma care nurse, community nurse or carer, should answer the following questions:

- What type of stoma does the patient have?
- What type of output comes from the stoma?
- Does the patient have full control of all his or her faculties (i.e. sight, hearing, mental ability)?
- Does the patient have good manual dexterity?
- What type of lifestyle does the patient have?
- What is the patient's peristomal skin like?
- How has the stoma been sited, is it in a difficult place?
- Does the patient have any preference, or is the patient happy to leave it up to the stoma care nurse's experience?

Stoma appliances can be divided into three specific categories reflecting the output of the stoma:

- Colostomy (formed to semi-formed stool)
- Ileostomy (effluent that is fluid and never formed)
- Urostomy (urine).

Appliances come in one-piece and two-piece systems (Figs 9.1–9.3) which can be transparent or, if the patient does not want to see the output, opaque. Many incorporate flatus filters, including, nowadays, ileostomy bags. Most ostomy companies make a range to suit most stomas and a few companies do a complete range to suit every eventuality. A one-piece appliance fixes over the stoma and has an integral adhesive area of hydrocolloid made from pectin, gelatin, cellulose polyisobutylene and sodium carboxymethyl-cellulose, which gives a hypoallergenic base. The integral adhesive may have an extra taped outer edge of micropore that helps to fit into body contours and folds and gives added security.

Two-piece appliances are made with a bag and base plate that fits over the stoma with a bag that clips on. The patient is thus able to change the bag as often as necessary without taking the base plate off the skin. This system is useful for patients from ethnic minorities who have to be clean prior to each prayer session, and enables them to have a clean appliance five times per day.

Colostomy

A colostomy may be formed in the sigmoid colon, descending colon, transverse colon and ascending colon, and the type of output will depend on the location of the colostomy. When a colostomy is situated in the ascending colon or in the area of the transverse colon in the hepatic flexure area, the output will be semi-solid. For these stomas the appliance needs to be drainable as the output will be needed to be drained off several times a day. Transeverse loop colostomies are often positioned in the right upper quadrant and are often temporary. Because of their size, these colostomies often present difficult management problems for the patient and the nursing staff, and suitable appliances can be difficult to find. Surgeons are encouraged by stoma care nurses not do this type of stoma unless really necessary. These colostomies are often done on the elderly patient who is debilitated and admitted during the early hours of the morning. Emergency surgery is necessary due to distal bowel obstruction and to resuscitate the patient. Postoperatively the stoma will be supported by a rod or bridge which will remain in situ for 5–8 days. The stoma will be large and elliptical and have a proximal and distal opening. The normal plan is to return the patient to theatre after whatever period of time is needed for them to become fitter. Unfortunately many return home but do not make sufficient recovery to come back for surgery and the community nurse and stoma care nurse are left to cope with a difficult, large transverse stoma. Sometimes for these stomas it is very difficult to find a suitable appliance which will enable patients to learn to care for themselves. Postoperatively an appliance that has an oval flange is the most useful and the adhesive area should be able to be cut up to 100 mm in size.

A colostomy placed in the descending or sigmoid area will have an output that is formed and easier for the patient to cope with. The appliance will be closed at the bottom and there will be a flatus patch at the top of the appliance to allow flatus to escape slowly and to stop the appliance ballooning, and it will incorporate a charcoal patch that helps to absorb odours. A new innovation to help with containing odour is the development of an additive to the colostomy appliance. This bullet shaped preparation is put into each new, clean colostomy appliance before use. It helps with odour both while the patient is wearing the appliance and when the appliance is removed. Innovations such as these can be especially helpful to patients who feel embarrassed about odour when visiting family or friends (Black 1999a).

Colostomy patients who find emptying and disposing of colostomy appliances difficult may benefit from a toilet disposal appliance. Although all appliances today are one use only, they are not toilet flushable. The appliance looks like a conventional appliance but has an inner lining. When the appliance needs changing, patients can remove the inner liner and flush it down the toilet. The remaining clean plastic bag can then be disposed of in the normal way.

Ileostomy

An ileostomy is formed in the right iliac fossa, often for inflammatory bowel disease. The output for an ileostomy, once it has settled down, is 350–800 ml of liquid effluent each day. For these stomas a drainable appliance is needed as the pouch needs to emptied up to six times in 24 hours. To allow the appliance to be sealed a clip or soft tie is needed. Here the ability and manual dexterity of the patient should be considered as to which will be the easier to use. When using the plastic clip to seal the appliance the pouch should only be wrapped around half a time and then clipped into place. Sometimes nurses wind the appliance end around the clip several times in the mistaken belief that it is safer that way, but this actually leads to the clip springing open and leakage occurring. Soft ties, which are similar to the ties used to do up rubbish bags, do, however, need to have the appliance wrapped around them four times or up to the shoulder of the appliance, for security and to avoid leakage.

Until 1997, filters on ileostomy appliances seemed impossible as the output was so fluid and the appliance would balloon up. The only way of relieving this was to go to the toilet and undo the clip at the bottom of the appliance and let out the flatus. This, of course, was not always convenient, and the patient would have to suffer with a large appliance that could show under the clothing, causing embarrassment. Now there are two ileostomy products that contain filters and which are available to patients on the drug tariff. These help with the problem of ballooning and work on similar lines to the filter on colostomy appliances and also have a charcoal insert that helps with dispelling odour. Although working on the same principle as colostomy filters, the filter needed significant technological thought to allow it to remain efficient in a wet condition and not block off.

Urostomy

A urostomy is raised in the right iliac fossa and needs an appliance that has a tap on the bottom. These appliances come in one- and two-piece systems and in transparent and opaque, although opaque has only recently become available. The urostomy appliance market is a small market – as few as 2000 urostomies are raised each year. The urostomy appliance incorporates a non-reflux valve or sleeve inside it to prevent back-flow of urine over the stoma and possible leakage, especially in the prone position. The drainage tap differs with each manufacturer and the patient should be assessed to find out which will be most suitable to use. The type of tap which can be easily flicked with the thumb or finger is the easiest for the patient who has problems with manual dexterity or who is paraplegic. The taps also have an indentation on them which indicates to the blind patient whether the tap is open or closed, so preventing mishaps. Urostomy appliances can have leg bags attached if needed which allows for added capacity, especially if the patient is unable to empty the appliance regularly (e.g. when travelling). At night for adult patients there is a night bag that can be attached to the appliance on the abdomen, allowing a greater collecting capacity (2 litres) and to save the patient from disturbed sleep due to having to get up and empty the appliance every 2–3 hours.

The appliances come with apertures of many sizes, from 10 mm to 100 mm. In hospital the appliance the patient has on from theatre is clear and cut to size and the appliance during the hospital stay is also clear. This enables the medical staff to continually observe the stoma and the output. On discharge the patient may have opaque appliances and the stoma may be settled enough to have pre-cut appliances. Today the hospital stay after gut surgery is very short – as little as 8–10 days – and the stoma will invariably not have settled down to the final size. It may therefore be necessary for the patient to have appliances that have a starter hole and are cut as needed. For some patients this is difficult due to problems with eyesight or manual dexterity. It may be necessary for the nurse to cut a supply of appliances before the patient leaves hospital. Alternatively, patients can receive pre-cut appliances via a dispensing appliance contractor (this is discussed further in community care, Ch. 15).

In deciding which appliance is correct for the patient several areas have to be taken into account. Patients with poor manual dexterity may not be able to manage a two-piece system and a one-piece appliance may therefore be more suitable. Also, if the one-piece system has an integral skin wafer there is only a single release paper to remove. Pre-cut holes eliminate cutting aperture size. Often the soft tie is easier managed than the plastic clip for drainable appliances. Patients with impaired or no vision will manage with pre-cut appliances and appliances with single release papers. A two-piece system may be easier as, once the base plate is in position, the pouch only needs to be clipped on regularly. The question of whether the appliance is transparent or opaque is not really of interest to patients with impaired vision and they tend to judge by the weight of the appliance whether or not it needs emptying. There is currently available on the European market an appliance which indicates to patients when it needs emptying. The pouch has lines and contact points on the outside which are programmed into a pager worn on the waistband or kept in the pocket in the way normal pagers are kept. The pager will bleep or vibrate when the stoma pouch reaches the pre-set level for emptying, so avoiding embarrassing accidents. For some patients this will be invaluable and the product should become available in the UK in 2000.

For patients with awkward stomas or those that have been placed in a difficult site, perhaps due to the fact that emergency surgery was needed and they were not preoperatively sited, an appliance with a flexible skin wafer such as a one-piece system might be the appliance of choice, although some of the recent two-piece systems are more flexible and can be used with

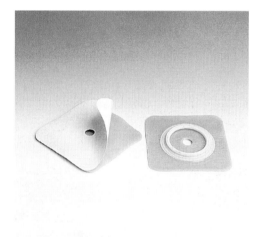

A

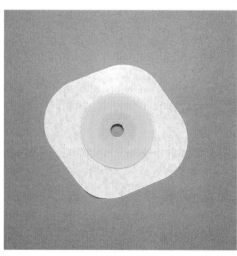

B

Figure 9.1 Two-piece flanges

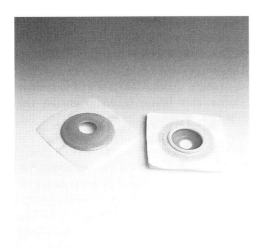

Figure 9.2 Convexity flange

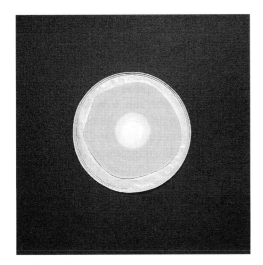

Figure 9.3 Stoma cap

awkwardly placed stomas. With some stomas, patients require a two-piece system that is going to be ultra safe, with no possibility that the pouch will come away from the flange. Two companies manufacture flanges and pouches that have a locking system that offers more security.

For patients with colostomies who are confident with their stoma management there is a system that enables the patient to be pouch free. However, there are limiting criteria. The patients must have an end colostomy and the output should be formed. This system is not suitable for any other type of stoma. The continent ostomy system

is a lubricated plug that is placed into the colostomy to seal it off (Plate 6). This is kept in place by clipping it to a base plate as in the two-piece system. Some time is needed beforehand to help the patient to become used to the plug, in the same way as one would need time, for example, getting used to contact lenses. Once used to the plug, the patient can wear it for up to 12 hours at a time. When the plug is taken out of the stoma, the build-up of faeces behind the plug is evacuated into a pouch connected to the base plate, or, with skill, the patient can learn to evacuate into the toilet. The original plug cannot be put back into the colostomy as the stalk of the plug has swollen to block stomal output. A new plug is needed for each use. Patient education is needed before using the plug and help should be sought from the stoma care nurse on the correct way to use the plug. For patients who find that there are occasions where flatus and a full stomal appliance could be difficult or embarrassing, the plug is an alternative.

For some patients with an end colostomy there is a way to empty the bowel daily so that there is no residual matter left in the colon. This is irrigation (Fig. 9.4). It can be offered as an alternative to wearing a colostomy bag. To do this regularly the patient must be motivated and have the uninterrupted use of a bathroom and toilet daily for at least 1 hour. There are strict criteria and the irrigation method should be taught by a stoma care nurse or other qualified practitioner in the comfort of the patient's own home. A specialised set to irrigate the bowel is needed and the few ostomy companies who make sets are usually able to give a complete starter set. Any replacement parts needed later are ordered via the prescription. The set comprises a 2-litre bag to hold the hypotonic solution (tap water) to wash out the bowel, tubing and a specialised silicone cone to conduct the water into the colostomy, a special extra-long bag known as a sleeve to conduct the water from the colostomy into the toilet pan, and a clip for the bottom of the sleeve. The patient sits on the toilet and applies the long sleeve to the stoma. The sleeve can fit as a one-piece item or a two-piece item. The bottom of the sleeve is put

The powdered form of karaya can be used on excoriated skin in the peristomal area to aid the adherence of an appliance.

Stomahesive® heralded a new era in stoma care and ostomy management. It was found to be non-allergenic and provides good adherence when used on stoma appliances and is tolerated on damaged and weeping skin (Black 1994a).

Night drainage bags are used by patients with a urostomy. The bag is connected to the body pouch allowing the patient to have a full night's sleep. Also available are leg bags. These connect to urostomy pouches to enable the patient to have a greater quantity collected, which can be useful when travelling or in situations that do not allow frequent emptying of the urostomy pouch.

Adhesive removers come in liquid form or in single, one-use sachets and help either to ease the appliance or to remove residue after the bag has been removed.

Skin barrier wipes are applied to clean, dry peristomal skin. Their action is to form a film on the peristomal skin, making a layer between appliance and any likely leakage from the stoma, thereby protecting the skin from excoriation. These wipes come in single, one-use sachets and contain alcohol to aid fast drying, so are not suitable to be applied to excoriated or broken skin. These skin barriers were nevertheless used around fistulas, but would sting. However, in 1999 a new preparation came onto the market as a skin protector around peristomal areas and around the skin of wounds and fistulas. Its form of application is either by multi-use spray or individual application by 'lollipop'. The advantage of this product is that it contains no alcohol, dries within seconds, needs only to be applied every 72 hours, and can safely be used on sore skin.

Cotton appliance covers were used frequently in the earlier days of stoma care as most of the appliances were not manufactured with soft body-side backings or needle film covers. Today, nearly all appliances are available with integral covers and the need for cotton covers is not so great. Covers absorb perspiration from the body and prevent the plastic appliance from feeling sticky and becoming stuck to the abdomen, especially in hot weather.

Belts are available from manufacturers for patients who feel that they need extra security in holding the appliance on. Patients who have a urostomy often feel more secure using a belt, and those with a colostomy or ileostomy also may feel that a belt gives added security. On two-piece appliances there are belt lugs to hook the belt into. For one-piece appliances where patients require a belt, a special plastic ring with belt lugs is available from manufacturers.

Abdominal supports and panty girdles which contain a custom made hole to accommodate the appliance – in consultation with the surgeon, GP or stoma care nurse – can be obtained either from the hospital appliance department or from a few of the stoma companies who have a girdle service. These belts and girdles are useful for patients who have a parastomal or incisional hernia where further surgical intervention is contraindicated.

DISPOSAL OF USED STOMA EQUIPMENT

Used stoma equipment in hospital is quickly and efficiently disposed off by placing it in yellow bags and sending to the incinerator. At this stage of their rehabilitation few patients have considered the implications of disposing of dirty appliances at home. A few may be aware that there is a collection service for used continence pads but this service does not apply to dirty stoma appliances. The disposal of used stoma appliances brings environmental concerns and when the patient returns home the used appliances are not classed as clinical waste but as household waste. With an estimated 80 000 ostomists in the UK, there can be an expected total output of at least 36 500 000 dirty stoma appliances each year. Today, with modern plastic production, appliances are classed as disposable, but not biodegradable, and they cannot be flushed via the sewerage system (Black 1987). In 1974 an HMSO report on disposal of difficult household waste stated (section 6):

The wider use of disposables in medical and nursing practice has increased the quantity of such wastes arising at home. These items are paper handkerchiefs, sanitary towels, babies' disposable nappies and stoma bags. A traditional and convenient way of dealing with some of these wastes was to burn them on the domestic fire or solid fuel burner. But the replacement of these forms of heating by other methods has removed this solution. Moreover burning at home is not suitable for the modern disposables made of plastic.

Section 10 states that further precautions for stoma bags are that they should be emptied down the toilet before the bags are wrapped for disposal. The long-term pollution problems arise not only from the stoma bags, but from appliances that are not emptied. Human excreta is a principal source of pathogenic organisms that are carried by water, food and insects. Soil contaminated by human excreta results in worm infestations, including hookworm. The sanitary disposal of human wastes is therefore necessary to eliminate contamination of the soil, water and food. In 1975 a report to the *British Medical Journal* (Plant & Devlin 1975) stated that while walking on a beach in Cleveland, UK, the authors had counted up to 30 used stoma appliances on the beach. How they arrived there, whether via the sea or local sewerage outflow, was a matter for conjecture.

Although some patients still lack indoor bathroom and toilet facilities, or have to share limited toilet and washing facilities with up to as many as 20 other families, generally improved living conditions and standards have also produced many difficulties in disposing of used stoma bags, with central heating and high rise flats causing specific problems. Black rubbish bags dropped down high rise rubbish chutes to a bin – which sometimes may not be there – will split open to display contents. Black rubbish bags put out overnight for next day collection can be torn open by fox or cat not only in the country but also in urban areas.

Urostomy appliances present fewest problems as they can easily be drained, wrapped securely in a plastic bag and put into the household rubbish. If patients do not have a supply of small plastic bags (such as the ones obtained at supermarkets), newspaper securely held is suitable, followed by disposal into the household rubbish.

Ileostomy appliances should be emptied into the toilet and rinsed through. It is not necessary to thoroughly clean the appliance. The easiest way to achieve cleansing is to hold the appliance at the front of the toilet bowl and pull the flush. The water will then pass through the aperture and out of the end of the appliance. The appliance is then wrapped and put into the household rubbish.

For colostomy appliances, the bottom of the bag needs to be cut and the contents shaken down the toilet. Again the best way of rinsing is to hold the appliance at the front of the toilet bowl and pull the flush. The appliance can then be wrapped securely in a plastic bag and put into the household rubbish.

Some patients who receive an appliance delivery service have, as part of that service, opaque plastic disposal bags sent to them specifically for the disposal of used appliances. For patients who cannot find suitable disposable bags, nappy sacks (sold by chemists and supermarkets for the disposal of dirty disposable nappies) serve the same purpose.

For some patients the disposal of their used appliance can seem an insurmountable problem, but discussion of the problem as part of the discharge planning and treating it as a normal procedure each day takes away the worry they feel about what will happen when they are at home.

10

The management of fistulas and large wounds

Fistulas and large abdominal wounds that can be associated with fistulas challenge the skills of the professional carer in protecting and keeping the surrounding skin integral and in the control of the effluent from the fistulas.

A gastrointestinal fistula is an abnormal communication between a part of the gastrointestinal tract and the skin (external), or between two parts of the gastrointestinal tract (internal), or between the gastrointestinal tract and another hollow organ (internal) (Fig. 10.1). Both internal and external fistulas can lead to rapid and life-threatening deterioration of the patient, with sepsis, malnutrition, electrolyte disturbance and ultimate dehydration, and 30 or 40 years ago these fistulas were associated with high mortality and morbidity and early definitive surgery had a mortality rate of over 50%.

Enterocutaneous fistulas can arise spontaneously from the stomach, duodenum, small bowel or large bowel. They most commonly arise from the small bowel or large bowel, from an underlying area of diseased bowel, or as complications of abdominal surgery when an anastomosis fails. Spontaneous intestinal fistulas can occur in association with Crohn's disease. Fistulas can be associated with radiation therapy prior to surgery when a bowel tumour is shrunk, or may be seen in diverticulitis.

Anastomotic failure leading to a fistula may be due to physiological or technical reasons. Physiological reasons may be ischaemia of the bowel, when too much of the blood supply to the bowel has been divided and the anastomosed

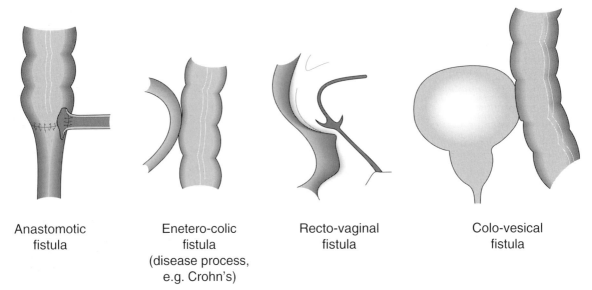

Anastomotic	Enetero-colic	Recto-vaginal	Colo-vesical
fistula	fistula	fistula	fistula
	(disease process,		
	e.g. Crohn's)		

Figure 10.1 Fistulas

ends are already ischaemic. If postoperatively the blood pressure falls after what is thought to be an anastomosis of healthy bowel, or the blood haemoconcentrates, the bowel may infarct and the dead piece of bowel will liquefy and ultimately perforate as an anastomotic leak. Prior treatment with steroids, as in Crohn's disease and ulcerative colitis, can lead to poor healing and the possibility that the anastomosis might leak. Diseases such as cancer and jaundice can also precipitate fistulas.

HISTORY

One of the earliest descriptions of a fistula is by Arateaus of Cappadocia, who in AD 39 incised an abscess in the right lower quadrant of the abdomen and this then resulted in an external fistula which subsequently spontaneously closed (Lichtman & McDonald 1944). In 1670, Thileus reported on a patient with biliary fistula (Horhammer 1916), and in 1735, Amyand described a faecal fistula in which the appendix had been incarcerated. Between 1900 and 1945, due to growing interest in fistula care, several authors published their work, and among these were Mayo & Schlicke (1941), Lichtman & McDonald (1944), and Lewis & Pewick (1933).

They found that most fistulas developed spontaneously, and that 58–80% were due to inflammatory disease and up to 19% due to postoperative complications.

Between 1945 and 1960, the opinion was that it was better to use conservative treatment initially before surgery was undertaken and surgery was only used if the patient was in the optimal condition. During this period it became understood that the most important factor in the welfare of the patient with a fistula was the resuscitation, which meant that dehydration, infection, shock, electrolyte imbalance and nutritional deficiency had to be corrected first. Even with the advent of antibiotics the overall mortality remained as high as 45% (Tenopyr & Shafiroff 1937).

From 1960 to 1970, the most common reason for fistulas was postoperative complications (Rinsema 1992). Primary conservative treatment remained the same and, with the improvement of the patient, resection of the fistula and bowel segment could be undertaken with an end to end anastomosis which was the procedure of choice (Nemhauser & Brayton 1967). Overall mortality was still high at 38–50%. Two developments that were responsible during this time for improved fistula treatment with conservative care were treatment using Chapman's protocol (Chapman et al 1964) and the evolution of parenteral nutrition (Dudrick et al 1968). Where parenteral nutrition was started within 48 hours of the recognition of the fistula, patients who received more than 2000 calories per day in this way showed a mortality of only 16%, whereas those patients who received 1000 calories per day or fewer had a mortality of 58%.

Between 1970 and 1980 surgical procedures became more aggressive and complicated and were often combined with chemotherapy and radiotherapy, raising the incidence of fistulas in people who had more advanced disease. Further improvements in intensive care of the fistula patient made conservative treatment more successful and the mortality dropped again to 15% and an increase in spontaneous closure of the fistula was also seen.

FISTULA CARE (Plates 7–9)

Skin and fistula care

Patients with fistulas or large abdominal wounds have to contend with a distinct body image problem just as much as patients with stomas do, and often these patients also have a stoma. When dressings are changed much of the patient's insides may be visible, depending on the depth of the wound and the layers that have broken down. In the case of an abdominal suture line dehiscing and opening, patients often find themselves looking at their own bowel, with both large and small bowel often protruding out. Large wounds and fistulas will be dressed with layers of dressing which become soaked very quickly and then begin to smell, which is distressing for both patients and their relatives. If there is effluent from the fistula or wound, especially small bowel effluent, it provokes excruciating pain and excoriation of the skin which also impacts unfavourably on the patient's quality of life. Gastrointestinal fistulas can take up to 12 weeks to repair, and patients can be in despair. Patients without hope are in a critical condition because hope is a necessary requirement for sustaining life. A positive approach to body

image change by patients who have large wounds or fistulas appears to be associated with improved healing. Cousins (1989) reports on the role played by various systems in bodily repair, suggesting that there is scientific evidence regarding the involvement of the psyche, nervous and endocrine systems in the body's healing process. Multiple factors affect the quality of wound and fistula healing, including psychological and physiological factors. Other obvious identified factors would be age, pre-existing conditions, infections and the state of the immune system (Laney 1969).

Control of the wound or fistula effluent and the protection of surrounding skin in large wounds is essential if successful treatment is to be carried out. Uncontrolled effluent onto surrounding skin leads to excoriation, pain, itching, infection and general deterioration of the patient. The continual problems of heavily soiled dressings, soiled night wear and bed clothes is disheartening for patient, carer and ward staff. The nature of the effluent from a fistula depends on its location. Proximal fistulas from the gastric, biliary, pancreatic or small bowel areas consist of activated juices and rapid digestion of the skin may occur with erosion to deeper layers. Colonic fistulas are less of a problem, as they have a less aggressive effluent and only a slow excoriation. The ultimate prognosis of the patient may be affected by adjacent intra-abdominal collections. Controlling the effluent diminishes these complications and when a fibrous channel develops spontaneous healing can occur, dependent on the site of the fistula and the functional ability of the distal bowel. Spontaneous closure can be expected in 8–12 weeks and if this does not occur then the fistula may be suitable for definitive surgery.

Historical aspects of fistula care

Many devices have been used and devised to stop or plug fistula sites to prevent excoriation of the skin and to control effluent. Formerly, neutralising or adhesive substances were often applied to the skin surrounding the fistula to form a protective layer over which the effluent could drain. Substances used included beef extract (Potter 1929), kaolin paste (CoTui 1930) and tannic acid (Dixon & Deuterman 1938). To block the fistula, such items as leather and wooden buttons, chewing gum and a double metallic button have been described (Dowd 1917). Because ordinary dressings, although absorbent, quickly become saturated and malodorous, suction devices were devised. One of the most famous was the Goldsmith cup (Goldsmith 1961, 1967). Another method was to support the patient on a Stryker frame (Patey et al 1946) (often used to nurse burns patients) to enable the fistula to drain. Modern stoma care provides a wide choice of materials useful for the care of large wounds and fistulas, both for the collection of effluent and for the protection of the skin. Problems related to high output fistulas can now be treated in a much simpler way, leading to hope for the patient of a complete recovery, and also giving an enhanced quality of life during the recovery period. Stoma therapists will have what is needed to protect and drain a large wound or will be able to advise on what to use and order. The stoma therapist can select the optimal treatment for this group of patients and either liaise with ward staff on the care needed or work with them when the appliances need changing. Care of these types of wounds has come to be seen as as much the remit of the stoma care nurse as stoma care itself (Black 1994b).

Skin barriers and pastes

In the 1950s, a skin adhesive called karaya, a natural absorbent rubber, started to be used, revolutionising stoma care and appliance management. However, some patients were found to develop allergies to karaya and liquid effluent caused problems with adherence and sometimes even washed it away (Turnbull & Turnbull 1991). Although karaya as a skin barrier sheet is still available, it has been superseded by Stomahesive®. In 1972, with the advent of Stomahesive®, a new era of stoma and wound care management started. Stomahesive® is a flat wafer made of gelatin, pectin, sodium, carboxymethylcellulose and polyisobutylene. It is generally resistant to

temperature and perspiration and much of the aggressive action of gastrointestinal fluid. It is tolerated by damaged, weepy skin and can remain in situ for up to 15 days. A comparative study of the properties of adhesives on the skin found that the nature of the adhesive was more important than the frequency of removal (Marks et al 1978). Current skin barriers which are available on the drug tariff are listed in Boxes 10.1 and 10.2.

Filler pastes

Filler pastes are used to fill uneven areas, crevices and hollows along and around wounds, fistulas and stomas to allow the appliance to have a flat, even surface on which to adhere. When uneven skin is evened up with paste, application of a skin barrier is more successful, thereby preventing leaks under appliances. If the skin is damaged or weepy, mixing a filler paste with Orahesive® powder helps the paste to adhere to the skin and also helps to protect the skin at the edges of the wound. The majority of filler pastes available on the drug tariff contain alcohol which helps with drying but can be painful when applied to open sore skin. Currently available filler pastes are listed in Box 10.3.

Appliances

There are several appliances available to stoma therapists which are ideal for wound and fistula care, and research and development departments

Box 10.1 Protective wafers	
ConvaTec	Stomahesive wafers
Coloplast	Coloplast protective sheets Coloplast protective rings
Dansac	GX-tra seals
Sims/Portex	Seel-a-Peel
B. Braun Biotrol	Skin protectors
Salts Healthcare	Cohesive seals Protective wafers
Hollister	Hollister skin barrier
Pelican	Pelican skin protector

<table>
<tr><td colspan="2">Box 10.2   Protectors and powders</td></tr>
</table>

ConvaTec	Orahesive powder
Coloplast	Comfeel protective film
	Comfeel barrier cream
Sims/Portex	Chiron barrier cream
	Derma-gard skin wipes
Salts	Peri prep skin wipes
Hollister	Skin gel
	Skin barrier

<table>
<tr><td colspan="2">Box 10.3   Filler pastes</td></tr>
</table>

With alcohol	**Without alcohol**
ConvacTec	ConvaTec
Stomahesive paste	Orabase paste
Hollister	Coloplast
Karaya paste and premium paste	Comfeel paste
Dansac	Pelican
Soft paste	Pelican paste
Simcare	
Seel-a-Peel paste	
Salts	
Stoma paste	

in ostomy companies are continually trying to produce the ideal product. Before the development of some of the products described below, a sump with suction was needed for most large wounds and fistulas. Even though appliances have improved considerably, occasionally the use of low pressure suction should be considered where the effluent is considerable and where there is difficulty in obtaining an efficient adhesion of an appliance. Sump suction may be indicated in the more complicated fistulas. It can be discontinued after fistulogram to exclude adjacent collections.

Wound manager (Convatec)

Indications for the use of this appliance are wound drainage management with postoperative draining wounds, fistulas, dehiscent wounds, Penrose drains and wounds with leakage around

the base of the drainage tube. The appliance allows continual observation of the wound, allows output to be assessed, adapts for wound size, shape and type of effluent output, enables cleaning and wound irrigation to be undertaken without the appliance being removed, and contributes to the patient's comfort and mobility.

Eakin fistula bags (Salts Healthcare)

These drainable appliances come in three sizes and have a cohesive interface seal. Cohesive combines adhesion with moisture-absorbing properties which ensures a good contact even when skin moisture is present. Digestive effects of ileal output upon the seal are diminished by the action of the soluble ingredients of the seal. The Eakin fistula tube drain is useful when drainage from the wound or fistula needs to be collected and measured separately from the wound output.

Hollister Wound Drainage System

The wound drainage system comes in three sizes with a hinged access cap and expandable side pleats to allow easy access for wound cleaning and dressing. The wide bore outlet allows for continuous drainage.

Coloplast Drainage Bag

This bag is ideal for all general drainage situations from wounds, fistulas, theatre and postoperative use. It has a large cutting area, skin-friendly adhesive seal with a microporos tape edging. It meets all the criteria suggested for postoperative drainage bags. There is now available a wound drainage bag that has a porthole door and allows for easy access to clean and irrigate wounds.

Simcare post-op classic

This bag was designed for large postoperative wounds and it reflects the need for continual monitoring of the wound. The adhesive flange is made of Seel-a-Peel and ensures a leakproof seal to body contours. Moisture is absorbed from the skin without breaking the seal down and it peels off with ease without breaking the integrity of the skin.

Convatec high output pouch

This pouch has been designed for patients who have high output from short bowel syndrome, jejunostomy, high output stomas, fistulas of the gastrointestinal tract or respiratory tract. Often the problem is high volume, malodorous, corrosive output. Frequent emptying and changing of dressings or inappropriate appliance can lead to sore, excoriated skin, increased risk of infection, poor quality of life and loss of confidence for patients, and are also time-consuming and costly in terms of nursing time and appliances used. This pouch has been designed to be used with the System 2 flange, enabling the flange to be left in situ for several days providing continuous skin protection, but allowing pouches to be clipped on and off as necessary. It has a wide-bore outlet tap giving provision for secondary drainage. It also has a flatus and odour filter which can be replaced without changing the pouch. The non-return valve prevents backflow of corrosive output, preserving the Stomahesive® skin barrier.

Many other ostomy companies make post-operative bags for small wound management with an adhesive cutting area up to 100 cm. But for large and difficult wounds and fistulas, any of the specialised wound care systems described above will give maximum comfort for the patient and greater convenience for the nursing staff.

NURSING CARE

Application of appliance

Management of fistulas begins with identification of the problem and identification of the type of output, followed by assessment and application of the correct type of appliance. Once the probable origin of the fistula and the type of output is established, the information will identify the possible risk of skin denudation and indicate the correct pouch selection and skin protection (Hannestead 1995).

Meticulous application of skin barriers and collective material and careful preparation of the skin are essential if leakage is to be overcome. Preparation and application should not be done in a hurry or in the middle of the night, when adequate time cannot be spent in the proper application of the appliances. After careful assessment of the wound and situation, the method of pouching is considered step by step and all the materials to be used are gathered together. Often, in order to keep the area dry, suction is needed whilst preparing the skin and wound, and if a high output fistula is present it may be easier to block the effluent output temporarily with a balloon catheter. Nowadays cleaning of the wound is done effectively with normal saline, and not with antiseptic. Antiseptics are activated by organic matter such as pus and wound exudate; they can also affect the blood supply in wound healing, and, in addition, bacteria are becoming increasingly resistant to antiseptics and their frequent use may contribute to bacterial resistance to antibiotics (Leaper et al 1987). The surrounding intact skin should be cleaned thoroughly with a mild soap and water. The use of soap as an astringent removes residual grease from the skin, allowing the appliance to adhere well. If necessary, the skin should be shaved. A skin protector such as Peri-Prep (Salts) or Cavilon (3 M) should be applied to an extensive area of the skin, including up to the wound edge. These preparations form a plastic skin which helps to protect against corrosive fluid and leakage onto integral skin. Next an application of paste mixed with Orahesive (ConvaTec) powder – used to absorb moisture from denuded skin and create a dry surface – is applied along the side of the wound or fistula. Skin barrier pastes and rings or strips are used to fill irregular skin surfaces such as scars, creases and skin folds and to protect the perifistula skin from effluent. When pouching, the paste makes a seal between the skin and the opening of the pouch. Over this an application of clear film such as Tegaderm (3 M) is laid up to the wound edge to help to keep the paste in place. It also acts as a waterproof barrier against corrosive effluent if leakage occurs. To enable the appliance to adhere well, while the wound or fistula is being prepared the appliance can be placed on a warm radiator prior to use. Using a template, cut a suitable sized opening into the appliance before removing the backing plate and place securely over the wound or fistula. The edges of the appliance, once in place, can be sealed again with Tegaderm to ensure complete security. Seal the end of the drainage bag or attach to a continual drainage bag.

Drug management

Drug management during conservative fistula treatment can be divided into two types:

1. Medication directed to decrease fistula output
2. Medication directed to septic complications.

In 1972 the substance somatostatin was isolated. It was shown to have potential in inhibiting gastrointestinal activity, but its disadvantage was that its short half-life necessitated continuous intravenous infusion. Since then, several analogues have been developed which can be administered subcutaneously and have a half-life of 90 minutes. The commonly used analogue is octreotide which is used as an adjuvant in the treatment of external gastrointestinal fistulas. The use of octreotide for the suppression of intestinal secretions and slowing the speed of intestinal transit also helps to increase water and electrolyte absorption and is valuable in the treatment of high output fistulas. The use of octreotide as an adjuvant medication to optimal conservative treatment of high output fistulas can reduce output considerably (to as low at 500 ml per day) and can speed the closure of the fistula after a short period of treatment. The use of somatostatin is recommended for patients if surgery is not advisable, if the fistula is life threatening, or if the fistula persists long term despite feeding by total parental nutrition.

H_2 blockers are often used to help control output from fistulas. They work on gastric, duodenal and pancreatic fistulas and inhibit, by competition, the stimulation of the H_2 receptors in the stomach by histamine, so consequently decrease the basic and stimulated gastric secretion and diminish pepsin production from the stomach. This can result in a daily reduction of output fluid from 2.5 litres per day to 0.8 litres.

Antibiotics

The correct place for antibiotics in fistula care is in treating septic complications, to which morbidity and mortality with fistulas of the digestive tract are usually related. The antibiotic regime should include antibiotics with a wide spectrum against colonic aerobes and anaerobes, including *Bacteroides fragilis.* The adjuvant use of gentamicin and metronidazole is advised perioperatively for 24 hours, with prolonged use only if there is uncontrolled sepsis, but the side-effect of antibiotic use – colonisation with resistant bacterial flora, nosocomial super-infections and allergic reactions – must always be remembered.

Successful pouching

Generally, a pouching system for fistulas should stay in place for 24 hours, and occasionally longer, depending on the placement of the fistula, the output and the degree of expertise in applying the pouch. It is rare that the first pouch will be 100% effective and this should be explained to the patient at the outset. Modifications are often necessary, such as a different pouch, a different template pattern or different adhesives. Explain to the patient, carer or ward staff that the pouch must be emptied regularly and that it should not be allowed to become more than one third full.

The advantages of a well-applied pouch are many. The skin is protected and the output contained. Cross infection and the sight and smell of the fistula are limited. There are no continual wet dressings, and accurate fluid output can be measured. The patient may be able to become mobile and have some hope, confidence and quality of life. Nursing time is saved and budgetary savings can be made. Once a pouch is in situ, care is still needed to make sure it does not overfill and that the appliance and adhesive are not wearing in the presence of alkaline proteolygic secretions which cause pain, discomfort, skin breakdown and bacterial colonisation. If leakage around the pouch is noticed it should not be padded, but the whole application removed and replaced again.

The management aspects of fistula care can stretch manpower, budgets and clinical skills. Patients with fistulas present stoma care nurses with challenges and opportunities to be creative and innovative in the care they give and in the teaching of the multidisciplinary team.

Case study: Millie

Millie had been admitted as an emergency to the surgical unit via A&E with acute abdominal pain. She was prepared for theatre. A laparotomy was undertaken and diverticular disease found. Because there was a perforation of the bowel from the diverticulum a Hartmann's procedure was done, resulting in a colostomy. Millie was told the news as soon as she was able to comprehend after the operation and the stoma therapist visited the next day. Millie was not too concerned about the colostomy as she had been looking after her mother who had had a colostomy 5 years previously – she was just relieved that the pain had diminished. Millie's recovery appeared to be uneventful until 4 days before discharge when the nurse noticed that the laparotomy wound was beginning to open. Steristrips and a dressing were put over it to hold the suture line. Unfortunately the wound dehisced and Millie had a large wound, 20 cm by 10 cm. Once the wound was clean the surgeon decided to let the wound heal by second intention and that the use of a hydrocolloid dressing would aid healing.

After discussion it was decided to try a new dressing, a hydrofibre dressing that used the main ingredient of the hydrocolloid dressing. This Hydrofibre™ (Aquacel®) dressing is designed for moderate to heavily exuding wounds as it absorbs exudate directly into the fibre.

Because exudate from wounds can contain enzymes, it can damage surrounding tissue and cause deterioration of surrounding skin. The Hydrofibre™ dressing can absorb up to 30 times its weight without losing its integrity, and it is composed of 100% sodium carboxymethylcellulose and therefore has no active ingredients.

The aim of treatment was to control exudate, maintain a moist wound environment, reduce pain levels and the use of analgesia, provide an atraumatic treatment regime, and promote healing. Over the next 3 weeks a considerable change in the size of the wound was seen and Millie was always keen to look and see how the size of the wound had changed. Once the wound was at an acceptable size for the community nurse to manage it was decided to send Millie home. She was coping with her colostomy and knew that once her wound had healed the surgeon would discuss the possibility of stoma reversal.

Millie returned to the outpatient department 8 weeks later. The wound was healed and although the skin was quite red and looked tender, she had no pain and in time the new skin would settle down. For Millie the use of a new hydrofibre had worked very well and had saved her from being transferred to the plastics unit for a split skin graft.

Adjuvant therapy

SECTION CONTENTS

11

Adjuvant therapy: radiotherapy

Colorectal cancer (see also Ch. 5) is the second commonest malignancy in the Western world. Each year in the UK, of the 25 000 new cases that occur, approximately half occur in the rectum. Surgery remains the primary treatment, with abdoperineal resection and permanent colostomy being required for most tumours in the lower rectum. If no further treatment is given after surgery, the tumour free survival rate is estimated to be as low 40%, with about 40% dying with uncontrolled pelvic disease. Recurrence may be local at the site of incision of the tumour (tumour bed recurrence), or it may be metastatic disease that has spread through the bloodstream, lymphatic system or peritoneal cavity. Some patients develop a further primary tumour in the colon, and although this is not a recurrence of the original tumour, it represents another focus of the disease. Careful surgery can do much to reduce the risk of local recurrence and adjuvant therapy for microscopic disease is of value. It is recognised that the use of adjuvant therapy such as radiotherapy (XRT) and chemotherapy (chemo) for patients who have colorectal cancer can substantially improve their overall prognosis.

RADIOTHERAPY

Radiotherapy (XRT) treats cancer by using high energy rays that destroy the cancer cells, while avoiding harming normal cells as much as possible. It is commonly used today in the treatment of colorectal cancer as there is evidence that the risk of recurrence is considerably less after XRT. It is suitable for treatment of cancer of the rectum, especially if it is thought that there may be cells in the pelvic area that are microscopically small. XRT is not normally given for cancer of the colon.

Neo-adjuvant radiotherapy (XRT before surgery) is sometimes given to patients whose tumour in the rectum is thought by the surgeon to be large or fixed. It reduces the size of the tumour and helps to make removal of the tumour at operation easier. The urologist may also recommend neo-adjuvant therapy for the patient who is to have a cystectomy, since it is now recognised that neo-adjuvant XRT reduces the staging of the tumour.

Radiotherapy can also be given for recurring secondary cancer, especially in the pelvic area, and to relieve pain.

Treatment planning

Once referral is made to the oncologist (who is the specialist in deciding how the XRT will be given), the patient will attend the radiotherapy department for a few visits before treatment commences. The simulator, a large machine, will take X-rays of the area to be treated and occasionally the patient will have a CT (computer-assisted tomography) scan, which gives a detailed picture of the inside of the patient's body. This is an important part of the XRT as it will show the area that is going to be treated. Marks are often drawn on the skin to aid the radiographer in positioning the patient accurately and defining exactly where the rays are going to be directed. The marks must be left on the skin during the treatment session, but can be washed off once treatment is completed. If indelible marks are needed so that the field of treatment is not lost, this is done with a tiny spot of ink, rather like a tattoo. It will be permanent. Treatment is not started until the staff are completely satisfied with the treatment plans. When XRT starts the patient is given instructions on care of the skin in the area that is going to receive treatment.

Treatment

Radiotherapy treatment is given by a machine called a linear accelerator which produces X-rays or gamma rays. XRT is not painful, but sometimes patients can feel very anxious at being on their own with just a machine. When the patient attends for treatment, the radiographer positions the patient, sitting or laying, and asks the patient to keep very still during administration of treatment. The administration is of a very short duration, but during it the patient is alone, although the radiographer can see the patient from the adjoining room and patient and radiogrpher can talk to each other if necessary. Patients who have a stoma may worry that the appliance will fill, overfill or leak and cause them embarrassment while they are undergoing treatment. The radiography staff should reassure stoma patients that there are facilities to change the appliance if necessary and patients should be able to empty the appliance before starting treatment if they wish (this is especially important for patients who have to have their treatment lying on their front).

As before surgery, it is now a legal requirement to obtain signed consent from the patient before starting the radiotherapy treatment. Patients may be asked to sign a form by the doctor who first advised XRT and this should be taken to the first appointment. If a consent has not been completed, it will be given to the patient at the first appointment

The oncologist decides what the appropriate treatment schedule for XRT should be. A course can be a single treatment or up to five treatments per week for 6 weeks, depending on a number of factors, including the aim of the treatment and the part of the body being treated. Some of the machines that deliver the treatment work faster than others and the length of treatment can be from 5 to 15 minutes. Hospital admission is not usually needed and patients travel to a designated centre, usually a cancer centre, on a daily basis. During the treatment the patient will have blood tests at various intervals and urine tests. X-rays or scans are also part of the routine while treatment is going on.

Side-effects

Radiotherapy is a localised treatment, which means that any side-effects will depend on the area of the body being treated. Every patient reacts differently, some experience mild discomfort and some may feel quite debilitated. XRT is not carried out until at least 6 weeks after surgery.

Tender skin

As the treatment progresses the skin in the field of treatment may turn red like a mild sunburn and the patient may experience tenderness and redness for 1 or 2 weeks after treatment has finished. The slight erythemous appearance of the skin is due to the X-rays affecting the tissues up to several weeks after treatment. The skin should not be washed in the area that is being treated and creams, deodorants, lotions, perfume or soap should not be applied. The materials from which they are made contain metals that may react to the treatment and make the skin even more sore. Boots's or Johnson's baby powder is suitable to use three or four times a day to soothe the skin and help any itching and also acts as a mild deodorant. Clothing should be loose and comfortable. The treated area should not be exposed to sunlight during treatment, or for some months afterwards, as the skin will burn more easily.

Tiredness

Towards the end of the course of treatment, patients often experience tiredness and lethargy, and this may last a considerable time, even after treatment has finished. It is important that the patient has as much rest as possible, although it is not unknown for some patients to continue with their employment all the way through their treatment.

Sickness

Nausea can usually be effectively controlled by antiemetics which will be given to the patient at the radiotherapy centre for the patient to take as necessary. Nausea and sickness are not experienced by all patients, and again it will depend on the part of the body being treated and the patient's susceptibility to the XRT.

Diarrhoea

For patients having XRT to the bowel or bladder there may be the problem of diarrhoea to cope with. Patients with stomas will find that they may have to change their colostomy appliance more frequently. In many cancer units the stoma therapist is part of the team and when patients come in for XRT the stoma therapist will be able to advise them on skin care and the use of an alternative appliance (such as a drainable one) while they are undergoing treatment. As cancer centres have a large catchment area, often covering several trusts, the stoma care nurse in the cancer centre is able to let the stoma care nurse in the patient's area know if the patient needs to have a different appliance or is experiencing difficulties while undergoing XRT. Likewise, when a patient is going to a cancer centre for treatment, the stoma care nurse looking after the patient can liaise with the stoma care nurse at the centre.

Sore mouth and throat

Normally this only happens if there is treatment to this area. But patients who are debilitated may experience a sore mouth or thrush and this can be treated with mouthwashes, drops or lotions that the radiographer or doctor will recommend. Teeth should be brushed with a soft toothbrush or dentures should be thoroughly cleaned and rinsed. Proprietary mouthwashes should not be used. Often a soluble aspirin, sipped, half an hour before meals can help.

Hair loss

Hair loss while having XRT is not usual, although some patients who have had XRT for bowel or bladder cancer may experience some hair coming out when they comb or wash their hair. This is not unusual when patients have been ill and undergone surgery, and is generally a normal reaction to the illness and/or surgery, and not an effect of the XRT.

Diet

Patients undergoing XRT are often tired and cannot be bothered eating regularly. Patients with a stoma may just be learning what foods suit them best, only to find that while undergoing XRT everything changes again. During treatment patients should drink plenty of fluid (of whatever they normally drink). A regular balanced diet should be eaten, taking into account the food that is suitable for the type of stoma that they have. Often the dietician will devise an eating plan especially for the debilitated patient. Sometimes, at the half stage of treatment, patients with a faecal stoma experience diarrhoea and advising them on suitable foods to eat may help. Other non-medical help are foods such as marshmallows and Jelly Babies, as they help to thicken the output. Often this is preferable to having medication prescribed.

Follow-up is 4–6 weeks after the end of treatment. The oncologist will discuss with the patient how the treatment has gone and what the continuing plan will be. Follow-up arrangements vary from patient to patient and this is discussed with the patient. Even though XRT is planned and delivered with the utmost care, sensitive parts of the body can be damaged. The bowel and bladder are particularly sensitive areas and XRT directed at either of these organs can cause damage to other associated organs, possibly leaving long-term changes. There is a 5% possibility that XRT may leave side-effects that affect the patient's lifestyle. While this may be unpleasant, it has to be weighed against the potential risk of the cancer progressing.

Stoma care nurses are well placed to help and discuss XRT with their patients when referral takes place. Once patients have been to the oncologist and know which regime they will be having, the stoma care nurse can discuss all the potential problems and explain how the treatment works and support this with the appropriate written information.

12

Adjuvant therapy: chemotherapy

Chemotherapy in cancer treatment means drug treatment using cytotoxic drugs systemically to destroy cancer. Unlike radiotherapy, chemotherapy can destroy not only the primary tumour but also the distant metastases. Systemic treatment can eliminate cancer or palliate metastatic disease. This can improve symptoms and quality of life. At least 25% of patients will have extranodal metastatic disease when they present with colorectal cancer. A large proportion will develop recurrent disease and only 35% will survive to 5 years. Cytotoxic drugs affect not only the cancer cells but also the normal cells.

Cytotoxic drugs are classified according to their role in the cell cycle (known as cell cycle specific). Cytotoxic drugs are cell cycle specific when cells are actively dividing and others are specific in a phase of the cycle of the cell (phase cycle specific). Cancer cells are most receptive to drug-induced damage when they are in a high growth fraction. This will depend on the type of malignancy and the stage of growth. Tumours that are in a high growth fraction and a short cycle are the ones most receptive to cytotoxic drugs (Holmes 1996).

In patients undergoing 'curative' surgery for colorectal cancer, it is expected that half will die before 5 years, predominantly with metastases in the liver. It has been shown that patients apparently having a curative resection have hepatic micrometastases. It is this that determines the probability of survival at 5 years (Finlay & McArdle 1986).

CHEMOTHERAPY

Administration

Chemotherapy is usually given in one of several ways:

- Orally as tablets or capsules
- By intravenous injection with a needle and syringe or by infusion
- By a continuous infusion
- Intramuscularly or subcutaneously.

The administration of chemotherapy can cause discomfort, especially in a vein, and this can be relieved by giving the drug slowly through a fast running intravenous fluid using a small cannula. The time scale for chemotherapy will be discussed with the patient by the oncologist and the regime explained. The regime will be specific to the patient and to the type of cancer the patients has. Treatments can be:

- Weekly
- Two, three or four times weekly
- Daily for short periods
- Continuously with a drip over a period of 1–5 days
- Continuously via an infusor system.

For some patients the administration of chemotherapy can be done over a period of a few hours as a day patient at a cancer centre in a special chemotherapy suite. For others, it may be necessary to be admitted to the ward for a 24–48 hour stay, or a 5 day stay within the cancer centre.

Side-effects

All patients react differently to chemotherapy, with some patients having no side-effects and others becoming quite ill.

Bone marrow depression is caused by the effect of the cytotoxic drugs on the bone marrow cells. Blood counts fall as the cells do not have time to reproduce properly, but will recover when there is a break from chemotherapy, which is why treatment regimes have a break between each dose. The administration of chemotherapy can be delayed if the blood count is too low and regular blood tests are taken to check for infection which will be rectified with antibiotics. If the patient is anaemic, a blood transfusion will be given.

If the white blood cells fall after the administration of chemotherapy the patient may experience a pyrexia, tiredness and the feeling of unwellness. Patients should be made aware that in this case they should contact the hospital immediately, as antibiotic cover may be needed.

If the platelets, which help blood clotting, fall, the patient may start to bruise easily for no apparent reason. Also there may be bleeding of the gums and nose. Patients should be told to minimise risk by taking extra care not to cut themselves and by using a soft toothbrush. If dental treatment is needed while on a course of chemotherapy, the centre should be contacted beforehand so that information about the current treatment can be given to patients for the dentist. Patients should also be told that they must report any blood in the urine to the doctor.

If red blood cells are affected by chemotherapy the patient may feel lethargic and look pale and feel short of breath. If this is due to anaemia, the patient will require a blood transfusion.

Hair

Contrary to general belief, not all chemotherapy causes the hair to fall out. Where hair loss occurs it is gradual, and the hair thins out. Much hair loss depends on the type of treatment that the patient is receiving and where the cancer is. With bowel cancer, patients notice a thinning of the hair but do not tend to lose it all. Once the drugs are finished the hair will regrow. It must be remembered that patients who have been ill and had surgery will lose some hair anyway.

Digestive tract problems

Patients undergoing chemotherapy will often complain of digestive upset, soreness of the mouth and gums (stomatitis), changes in taste and smell, nausea and vomiting, diarrhoea and constipation.

Avoiding hot and spicy food, acidic food and reducing alcohol and smoking while undergoing chemotherapy will help with some of the side-effects. Redness and soreness of the gums, bleeding gums and ulcers are often side-effects of chemotherapy. These can be helped by using mouthwashes from the chemist and cleaning the teeth with a soft brush. Sucking an ice cube while chemotherapy is given may reduce the risk of mouth upsets.

Due to the type of drugs used in chemotherapy the patient may experience a disruption of taste and smell. Often ordinary water will taste metallic and patients generally experience a metallic taste in their mouths which affects their appetite. Sucking a strongly flavoured sweet at the time of injection may help to allay the taste change or keep it to a minimum. Small meals may be more appealing than normal sized ones, and low fat meals are often easier to tolerate, with dry crackers or toast helping with nausea. Carbonated drinks can help settle the stomach, but patients with stomas should take these with caution as flatus may be hard to control and cause continual inflation of the appliance.

Diarrhoea can occur with some of the drugs administered and can cause more problems for the patient with a stoma. Medication may help, but marshmallows or Jelly Babies help to thicken the output and the lemonade drink 7UP helps with diarrhoea. Patients with an ileostomy who undergo chemotherapy should drink as much as possible to avoid dehydration. Constipation may occur while treatment is progressing and laxatives may be prescribed. Often patients with a faecal stoma who have chemotherapy find that the stoma swells and feels very tender and sore for a few days. Reassurance and an explanation of how chemotherapy works is enough to put patients' minds at rest.

Work and play

A few patients manage to continue to work throughout their treatment regime or between courses, but activity should be limited and plenty of rest taken. Often the effect of the treatment is not felt until after two or three courses. Any holiday plans should be discussed with the oncologist as treatment courses should not be broken. If the doctors know that the patient wishes to go away, treatment can be planned around these dates. Long periods in the sun should be avoided while on certain chemotherapy regimes. If vaccinations are needed for a holiday the advisability of this should be checked with the oncologist first.

A normal sex life can continue while on treatment, but often the patient feels too tired and is trying to tolerate the side-effects of chemotherapy. It is very important that pregnancy is avoided whilst either partner is having chemotherapy and a reliable form of contraception should be used. Sterility may occur in men and may be permanent or temporary. Sperm banking should be considered and discussed with the oncologist before starting treatment. Women may also find they become sterile, and this also may be temporary or permanent. Menstruation may stop or become irregular during chemotherapy and it is advisable to avoid pregnancy for a year after treatment has finished.

DRUGS USED IN CHEMOTHERAPY

The most commonly used chemotherapeutic drug used in the management of colorectal cancer is 5-fluorouracil, a fluorinated pyrimidine. Until recently, results from studies investigating the effects of different doses of 5-FU have been disappointing, leaving surgeons and physicians divided in their views of whether adjuvant chemotherapy and radiotherapy have a role to play in the management of colorectal cancer (Knowles & Jodrell 1997). Recently published studies have shown that the use of 5-FU with levamisole and 5-FU with folinic acid reduces the relapse rate by 40% and mortality by one third in patients with node positive colorectal cancer (Slevin 1996). 5-FU with either levamisole or folinic acid has some toxicity, giving rise to nausea, mucositis, diarrhoea and lethargy, which can be helped by antidiarrhoeal drugs and antiemetics. Adjuvant chemotherapy has a role in the treatment of colorectal cancer for patients who have a tumour staging of Dukes C, but its use in tumours staged at Dukes B is not yet established.

There is some evidence to show that the use of monoclonal antibodies such as (mAb) 17-1A (Panorex) may possess antitumour activity against cancer cells in the resting phase and against cells resistant to conventional chemotherapy. At present this treatment is only in the trial stage. Irinotecan has been used and has shown it causes shrinkage in the cancer in a proportion of patients whose cancers who have are resistant to a 5-FU and folinic acid. Campto® (irinotecan hydrochloride trihydrate) is a new drug in the treatment of colorectal cancer that can offer good quality palliative care for many colorectal cancer patients with metastases who have not responded to a 5-FU regime. Campto originates from the Chinese tree *Camptotheca acuminata* and its parent drug, camptothecin, was isolated in 1957. The response rates are 11–23%, which can be considered to be low, but patients receiving this treatment are patients who do not benefit in terms of survival (Massey 1997).

CLINICAL TRIALS

Research into new ways of treating colorectal cancer is being undertaken all the time. No current treatment results in a cure and many hospitals take part in these trials. If a new treatment appears to be better than a standard treatment, trials will be carried out to compare the new treatment against the best standard treatment currently available. This is known as a controlled trial. So that the treatments can be compared accurately, the patient's type of treatment is randomised by computer. If doctors make the randomised choice themselves, an element of bias, albeit unintentional, can come into the trial. In a randomised trial some patients receive the best standard treatment while the others receive the new treatment.

Patients will be asked to participate in a trial at centres where there is a trial going on. The trial will have been approved by the local ethics committee and the patient is asked to give informed written consent and is given a patient information sheet explaining all about the trial. At any stage the patient may pull out of the trial without affecting his or her continuing care.

Trial CRO7

This Medical Research Council trial was to address the question: should all patients with operable rectal cancer receive a preoperative short course of XRT, or is it better to give postoperative XRT only to those patients with involved margins following surgery? Over a 3-year period, 1800 patients needed to be recruited into the trial. A key factor is to keep the time between preoperative XRT and actual surgery to a minimum, preferably within 1 week.

AXIS trial

This trial aimed at recruiting 4000 patients who had been randomised for portal vein infusion therapy, with a further 748 being randomised to receive radiotherapy.

CRO5 trial

This trial aimed to compare the de Gramont regimen of 5-FU/folinic acid given via intravenous and intrahepatic arterial procedures. Recruitment was 312 patients.

CRO6 trial

This three arm trial is comparing the standard de Gramont bolus and infusion regimen of 5-FU/folinic acid to the Lokich regimen of continuous infusion of 5-FU and a regimen bolus of Tomudex (Zeneca). Nine hundred patients are needed for statistical analyses.

CLASICC trial

This trial compares laproscopic versus convential surgery in colorectal cancer. Patient numbers are 1000, by 14 surgeons in 11 centres. From this trial patients can be entered into the AXIS trial or the QUASAR trial.

QUASAR trial (Quick And Simple And Reliable)

This trial is designed to provide evidence of the true value of different adjuvant chemotherapy regimens among different types of patients. It aims to randomise a very large heterogeneous group of colorectal cancer patients between chemotherapy and no therapy, and also randomising patients between the most promising chemotherapy regimens. The information on a few thousand randomised patients will then help guide the treatment of many hundreds of thousands of future patients.

There is simple eligibility to the trial: resected colorectal cancer, no distant metastases, no 'definite' contraindications to chemotherapy. The question to be asked at randomisation is if the indications for chemotherapy are 'clear' or 'uncertain'. The decision as to whether the patient is to be in the clear or uncertain arm of the trial lies with the doctor and patient.

Patients entering the 'clear indication' arm will be randomised between:

- 5-FU + high dose folinic acid + levamisole
- 5-FU + high dose folinic acid + placebo
- 5FU + low dose folinic acid + levamisole
- 5FU + low dose folinic acid + placebo.

Those patients randomised into the uncertain arm will have:

- Chemotherapy as for 'clear' indication
- No chemotherapy.

Patients who enter the uncertain arm and are randomised into 'no chemotherapy' will need support and reassurance from the medical staff and either the stoma therapist if the patient has a stoma, or the colorectal nurse, to support them in understanding that they are not considered not worth treating but that, with their informed consent, they were prepared to enter the trial and were randomised in this way.

This trial had effectively nearly reached its target, with 5250 patients recruited, and its target for chemotherapy, but needs more patients to be randomised into the uncertain arm for chemotherapy. The rate of recruitment had been slow into the uncertain arm, but was beginning to increase.

The treatment of colon cancer has been transformed over recent years from a therapeutic desert into one of the most innovative and fast moving areas of laboratory and clinical cancer research (Slevin 1996).

13

Assessment and management of stomas, fistulas, catheters and drainage tubes in palliative care

In considering the whole person in palliative care there needs to be an integrated approach to the management of stomas and their problems, the difficulties that fistulas can bring and the general care of catheters and drainage tubes. Besides the confrontation of mortality for these patients and their families, there is the problem of complex physical symptoms that may have given rise to palliative stoma surgery with complications that lead to fistulas. There may be a need for wound drainage tubes and often the need for urethral or suprapubic catheters. With these extra problems, the existing psychological and emotional problems already encountered, leading to a poor quality of life, become a challenge for the palliative care team.

Care then depends on an interdisciplinary approach with a mutual respect for all team members and good communication enabling the patient, where possible, to be involved in any decision making about care and treatment. Cousins (1989) suggests that there is scientific evidence of the role played by the various systems in bodily repair and healing. He reported the evidence regarding the influence of the psyche, and the nervous and endocrine systems on the body's healing process and concluded that positive emotions are associated with improved wound healing. Psychoneuro-immunology researchers believe that positive emotions alter the production of certain hormones, neurotransmitters and opioids that can interfere with the various steps in the healing process.

Specialist nursing knowledge such as that of the stoma therapist in the assessment and management of palliative patients with stomas, fistulas and drainage tubes represents an essential contribution to the palliative care team. The research of Dunkel-Schetter (1984) indicates the importance of providing the right amount of information to the patient and the importance of that information coming from an expert.

PALLIATIVE CARE AND THE MANAGEMENT OF STOMAS AND FISTULAS (Plates 7 and 8)

The main problems of palliative care patients with stomas that will require specialist input are:

- Nausea
- Vomiting
- Abdominal distension
- Constipation
- Diarrhoea
- Nutritional difficulties
- Pain
- Difficulties with stoma appliances
- Emotional and psychological difficulties.

Dealing successfully with one or many of the physical problems has often been seen to alleviate emotional and psychological problems, leading to a raised morale and hope that is not necessarily associated with recovery or cure.

The principal symptoms of gastrointestinal malignancy are usually due to recurrence of the tumour, blood loss through erosion of a vessel by a tumour, or obstruction by tumour bulk, and it may be necessary for the patient to undergo palliative surgery for a stoma or bypass of the tumour. Patients will often be debilitated prior to surgery due to weight loss and may have many of the symptoms listed above.

There will be body image problems associated with a stoma or gastrostomy, often with further weight loss, and possible sexual difficulties with spouse or partner. A stoma may only give short-lived relief of symptoms. Patients who have come into hospital from palliative care in the community may fear that they will not be able to go home again. Some patients may be unable to participate in any decision making about palliative surgery, yet the short term gains may make an invaluable contribution to a patient's limited quality of life.

Pain, nausea and vomiting are managed by pharmacological intervention by the palliative care team but often analgesia can cause intractable constipation, contributing to nausea and vomiting. If the patient is able to take oral input, raising the fluid intake is important, and larger amounts of water help with possible dehydration. Large quantities of tea and coffee (which both contain caffeine) will aggravate constipation and contribute to dehydration. If the patient is able to eat, raising dietary fibre may help. Foods high in natural fibre are porridge oats, Shredded Wheat, root vegetables and brown bread. Kiwi fruit (one per day) is an excellent fruit to use to help relieve constipation whether the patient has a stoma or not. If the patient is unable to eat, an enema or suppositories via the colostomy may help. Glycerine suppositories may be put down the stoma but they must be held in the stomal opening for at least 20 minutes to allow them to dissolve, otherwise the stoma will expel them immediately they are inserted. Alternatively, an arachis oil enema may be instilled via the colostomy, preferably in the evening, immediately before retiring. Turning the patient on to the right side to sleep allows the oil to penetrate across the transverse colon and down to the ascending colon. This may need to be repeated on the next evening. (Note that anyone with a nut allergy should not be given an arachis oil enema or administer one.)

Diarrhoea is often a problem, especially if patients are undergoing chemotherapy, and it can be distressing to continually have leaking appliances leading to sore and excoriated skin. If the patient is able to have oral intake, again a high fibre intake will help to alleviate diarrhoea. White cooked rice and even rice water are useful, along with stewed apple and smooth peanut butter. Marshmallows and Jelly Babies also are useful to help stop diarrhoea, as is the old-fashioned remedy of arrowroot in a little warm milk taken orally. Medication may have a number of undesirable side-effects on stoma patients because of the effect the drugs may have on the gastrointestinal function. Some patients need medication to modify bowel transit time and loperamide, methylcellulose, isphagula and sterculia are suitable. Medication taken for long standing illnesses may cause problems (e.g. antibiotics, which cause diarrhoea, and tricyclic antidepressants, which have an anticholingeric effect on the gut causing constipation and faecal impaction (Black 1994c).

STOMA APPLIANCES

Many of the difficulties that palliative patients with a stoma experience are difficulties with appliances. Problems may occur due to weight loss causing the appliance to fit incorrectly and the aperture to be the wrong size, leading to skin soreness. Sometimes weight loss can lead to the stoma retracting below the skin surface, causing leakage onto the skin. To help alleviate these problems, patient and stoma and appliance need to be assessed carefully and appropriate changes made. If weight loss is the contributing factor, changing the appliance from a two-piece to a flexible one-piece appliance that will fold into the body contours may help. Checking the aperture size of the original appliance may show that the aperture needs resizing. If the stoma has retracted below the abdominal surface and the output leaks under the flange onto the skin, and surgery for resiting the stoma is not feasible, the use of stoma appliances with convexity may be the solution. Convexity should only be used under expert guidance as incorrect use can damage a stoma.

A transverse colostomy is often done as an emergency in acutely ill or palliative care patients as a short-term measure and as a quick surgical procedure to relieve obstruction. Unfortunately, prolapse of the transverse colostomy occurs in about 20% of patients and can be an extremely difficult management problem for patient or carers. Often large postoperative stoma bags are required, or specific specialist appliances, and the stoma therapist is the ideal person to advise the team, patient and carers on these.

FISTULA MANAGEMENT (Plates 7 and 8)
(See also Ch. 10)

A particular challenge of caring for patients with large wounds and fistulas is ensuring that the skin surrounding the wound is protected from effluent and that the effluent is kept under control. Excoriation of the skin, itching, pain, infection and general deterioration of the patient's condition are possible consequences of allowing the continual discharge of effluent. Patients with large wounds or fistulas have to contend with a distinct change in body image and it is also distressing for such patients, at dressing changes, to catch sight of their internal organs. Moreover, if a suture line dehisces and opens, patients may find their intestines extruding. When the nutritional status of a palliative care patient is compromised, if recent surgery has been done, this may be one of the added complications. The odour from these wounds can be offensive and the application of continual layers of wet dressings each day exacerbates the problem.

The location of the fistula will in part determine the type of effluent produced. Fistulas approximate to the gastric, biliary, pancreatic or small bowel areas exude corrosive juices. Colonic fistulas are less of a problem and their output is less damaging.

Today, a wide range of materials is available to ensure adequate collection of effluent and to give protection to the skin and in doing so endeavour to give the patient a better quality of life. The stoma therapist is in an excellent position to advise and show the palliative care team how to use and apply these items, all of which have derived from stoma care appliances (Black 1995d).

Filler pastes contain numerous components, including gelling and film forming agents. Ethanol may be included to help them set. The paste is applied to fill cracks or gullies to make a level surface on which to apply a fistula bag or stoma appliance. Because the majority of stoma pastes contain alcohol to help them set, this can cause distinct pain if applied to excoriated skin.

Skin barriers are made from karaya gum or today, more often than not, Stomahesive® or hydrocolloids. The introduction of Stomahesive in 1972 had a major impact on stoma and wound care management. The hypoallergenic nature of the wafer reduces skin irritation. Such products can be left in situ for 15 days or more and can be integral to the appliance or on a separate flange (Marks et al 1978).

There are several appliances which are ideal for wound and fistula drainage (see Plate 15). As a guide, an appliance should be used when the output of the effluent is greater than 100 ml in 24 hours.

When deciding on the type of appliance to use the following factors should be taken into consideration:

• Wound size
• Type of wound
• Amount of exudate
• Individual patient needs.

Meticulous preparation of the skin in fistula care is of vital importance if the skin is to be protected. Applying a fistula bag takes time and should not be rushed or the whole object of the exercise is wasted. After careful assessment of the wound or fistula the chosen method should be considered step by step and all the appropriate materials gathered together. Invariably it will need two pairs of hands to complete a successful job. Suction apparatus may be required while cleansing and preparing the fistula if there is excessive exudate. Alternatively the fistula can be temporarily blocked using a balloon catheter. Normal saline is the currently accepted solution for cleansing. The surrounding intact skin should be thoroughly cleaned with a mild soap and water and, if necessary, the area shaved (Leaper et al 1987). It may be necessary to fill any gullies with paste. The paste is taken up to the sides of the wound and the paste and skin barrier are covered with a vapour-permeable dressing film to keep both in situ. The film dressing should be taken to the edge of the wound to provide protection for the healthy skin.

All fistula bags are made so that they can be cut to size and shape. Most have a central hole as a point to start cutting. The fistula or wound should be assessed regularly to ascertain changes in aperture size and these made accordingly, making a new template each time. The appliance is put over the film dressing and the end sealed with either a stoma bag clip or attached to a continuous drainage bag if the fistula is a high output fistula.

The management of large wounds and fistulas is challenging and time-consuming and a system will hopefully stay in place for 24 hours. It is rare that a fistula pouch applied for the first time will be 100% effective. The importance of maintaining the integrity of the skin surrounding the fistula cannot be over-emphasised. Of equal importance is that the patient has confidence in the staff and the system being used.

MANAGEMENT OF DRAINAGE TUBES AND CATHETERS

Palliation may also involve the insertion of catheters and drainage tubes or stents to create artificial lumens or to bypass obstructions. These tubes may go into the pancreas, biliary, oesophageal and kidney areas, or they may be tubes such as gastrostomy or jejunostomy which will be used for feeding purposes. The output from the upper gastrointestinal areas can be exceptionally corrosive if allowed to come into contact with the skin and care must be taken to protect the surrounding skin where the drainage tubes arise. Initially, after placement of the tube, an ordinary dressing is placed over the area to keep the tube in place. Often leakage will occur around the tube and the skin will start to become red and sore. Every time there is a leakage the dressing must be removed, the skin washed thoroughly to remove enzymes on the skin, and a new dressing applied. This may become extremely upsetting for the patient, and ways to reduce the continual replacement of dressings should be found. Here the stoma therapist will have a whole range of skin protectors to protect the skin around the tube. Skin barriers may be used as a one-piece or two-piece application and will protect the skin from exudate. The efficiency of skin barriers can be assessed by the ability to resist heat and perspiration and to protect the skin from the corrosive action of the exudate.

A skin barrier is easier to apply in the form of a flat square that can be cut to the appropriate size and shape and may be left in situ for up to 15 days. Manufacturers' instructions should be followed carefully in order to ensure the safe use of all products. Occasionally it may be necessary to apply a stoma bag over a drainage tube such as a nephrostomy tube to keep the patient dry.

Catheters (e.g. suprapubic) may need to have a skin protector placed around the base at skin level to stop leakage spilling onto the skin. Secretions which often occur around the catheter site can be removed by bathing with soap and water. Over granulation of the tissue at the catheter site can be removed with the use of silver nitrate.

Meatal cleaning around urethral catheters should take place where the catheter enters the body. Increased secretions occur with the use of urethral catheters due to the irritation of the urothelium. The secretions form crusts which, when removed, form areas of exposed damaged tissue that can be prone to bacterial colonisation which can ascend into the bladder. Roe (1993) recommends cleaning with soap and water and a clean cloth each time. The frequency depends on the amount of secretions, but twice a day is usually sufficient.

It is clear that there is a need for the specialist skills of the stoma therapist in the palliative care team and that they are crucial to the support of the patient, carers and nurses. The challenges and needs of the palliative care patient are often complex, and surgery and surgical innovations have extended treatment possibilities for patients who may be in the advanced stages of malignant and non malignant disease, yet may cause further management problems. In giving the patient hope and a better quality of life the team can make a positive difference within the limitations of advanced illness.

Care in the community

SECTION CONTENTS

and be able to manage leakage and odour and ways of living with a stoma. If patients have not achieved confidence and competence in practical care, it is unlikely that they will adjust psychologically (Mead 1994).

Planning towards discharge will have assessed each individual's requirements and concerns, some of which have already been mentioned in this chapter. A planned programme will have been started from the first postoperative day, although the patient at this stage is merely a spectator and not a participator. For the patient to move from spectator, to participator, to self-carer takes a number of well-defined practical steps. Figure 14.2, 10 steps to self-care, highlights how care moves from the nurse to the patient. This time-frame allows the patient to progress through each stage, usually on a daily basis until discharge. Wilson & Desrisseaux (1983) suggest that by careful planning and recording of any teaching that is undertaken, unnecessary over-teaching and wasting of valuable time is avoided. Logical planning helps the patient to understand the current process and what the next step might be.

Orem's self-care deficit nursing theory

Nursing theories or conceptual frameworks are, in the West, considered to be the core of nursing science, as they frame the domain of nursing as a discipline within the concepts of person, environment, health and nursing. A suitable conceptual framework for the stoma patient, evaluated for its applicability of knowledge, willingness and skill, is Orem's self-care deficit nursing theory (SCDNT) (Orem 1991, Tomey & Alligood 1998). Conceptual models provide different ways of thinking about nursing and address the broad metaparadigm concepts that are central to its meaning. The central assumption of Orem's framework is that people require nursing care when their needs for care exceed, or can be predicted to exceed, their own ability to meet these needs (Orem 1991). Orem's theory views the person as a human being who functions biologically, socially and symbolically and as an

agent who can meet his or her own self-care needs. The theory is described as three related theories:

1. Self-care is described as a practice of activities that maturing and mature persons initiate and perform within time-frames, on their own behalf, in the interests of maintaining life, healthful functioning, continuing personal development and well-being.
2. The theory of health care deficit describes and explains why people can be helped through nursing.
3. The theory of nursing systems describes the relationships that must be brought about and maintained for nursing to be produced.

A helping method is a series of successive actions which, if performed, will overcome the limitations of the person at that time due to their ill health. These actions help to regulate the patient's own functioning and development or those of their carer. The methods are used in combination or individually by the nurse in the care of the patient while the patient's health-associated actions are limited. These actions are:

- Acting or doing for another
- Guiding and directing
- Providing and maintaining an environment that supports personal development
- Teaching.

Orem (1991) describes three levels of nursing systems: wholly compensatory, partly compensatory and supportive–educative. In using the 10 steps to discharge for stoma patients (Fig. 14.2), the patient and nurse move through the three stages together. While the nurse takes care of and changes the stoma appliance in the early postoperative days because the patient is unable to perform actions or control actions, the system is wholly compensatory. When the patient starts to share the care of stoma management under the nurse's supervision the system is partly compensatory. Once the patient is able to undertake self-management of the appliance and change the appliance, the nursing system becomes supportive–educative.

There is much research on teaching self-care to individuals with a variety of diseases using

The
Hospital

STOMA APPEARANCE
AND FUNCTION

UNIT No.

SURNAME
(block letters)

FIRST NAMES

D.O.B.

WARD

Patient Label

Type of stoma _____ Consultant _____

Special Instructions

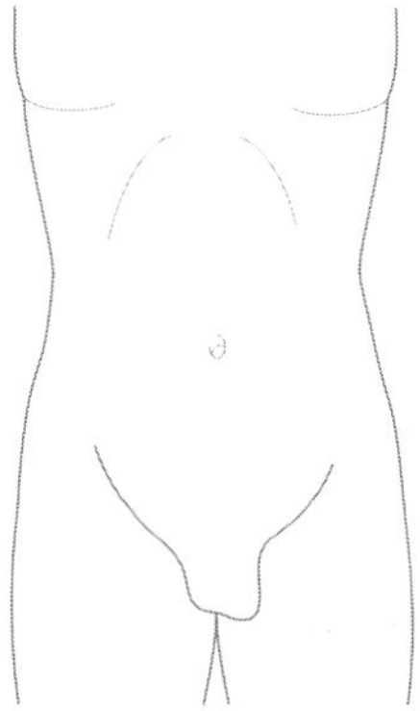

Stoma site
Indicate:
Skin creases
Scars
Hernias

Post-op day	Time	Stoma colour	Appearance e.g. oedematous flush, retracted	Condition of peristomal skin	Stoma action e.g. flatus, liquid, formed stool, constipated	Signature
1						
2						
3						
4						
5						
6						
7						

Figure 14.1   Discharge planning: reviewing the stoma

1. Teach patient to remove and re-attach clip to bottom of bag.

Met/Not met

If not met, comments:

6. Teach patient how to measure their stoma and why.

Met/Not met

If not met, comments:

2. Teach patient to empty bag.

Met / Not met

If not met, comments:

7. Show patient a selection of appliances and, with guidance choose one suitable for their needs.

Met / Not met

If not met, comments:

3. Teach patient re.equipment required to change appliance.

Met / Not met

If not met, comments:

8. Teach patient how to apply new bag.

Met / Not met

If not met , comments:

4. Teach patient how to remove bag from skin.

Met / Not met

If not met, comments:

9. Instruct patient how to dispose of used bags.

Met / Not met

If not met, comments:

5. Teach patient how to wash and dry stoma and surrounding skin.

Met / Not met

If not met, comments:

10. Teach patient the use of accessories.

Met / not met

If not met, comments:

Appliance in use

Manufacturer	Closed / Drainable	Opaque / Clear	Code No.

Figure 14.2   Discharge planning: teaching patients self-care

the core concepts of SCDNT, particularly in the areas of pain management and oncology. Other areas suitable for the application of Orem's theory and concepts are psychiatry and mental health. Orem's theory and concepts for patients and families who are managing the side-effects of chemotherapy and radiotherapy have also been applied to stoma patients undergoing adjuvant therapy.

The stoma care nurse will liaise with the ward staff in regard to the date of the patient's discharge. The ward will normally take care of transport arrangements, any social service input and, if necessary, arrange for a district nurse to visit. In the case of a paediatric patient, arrangements for the paediatric liaison team and health visitor will be made by the ward. In some areas the hospital stoma care nurse continues care through to the community and will arrange with the patient a suitable day and time to visit him or her at home within a week of discharge. Very few patients will refuse a home visit and some are under the misapprehension that the stoma care nurse will visit daily.

Wade (1989), in her research study of stoma care nurses and their patients, found that 93% of patients in districts that had a stoma care nurse had received at least one visit from the stoma care nurse at the time of interview. In non stoma care nurse districts only 7% of patients had received a visit from a stoma care nurse. Stoma care nurses were asked about their planning of community visits and how often they visited patients. Over the first year the patient could receive anything from a single visit to 10 visits, depending on the nurse's policy. In five of the districts where interviews took place the stoma care nurses stated that they visited within 48 hours of discharge. In areas where there was no community stoma care nurse, 82% of patients had been visited by a district nurse. Unfortunately, some patients in non stoma care nurse areas said

that the visit by the district nurse was unhelpful and that the nurse did not seem to know anything about stomas. In non stoma care districts 46% of stoma patients had been visited by a company stoma care nurse and most found this useful. One patient, though, objected to the company nurse pushing her own company product and the wrong type of appliance as well.

Patients' perceptions of who has been of most value to them on their discharge show that they value the spouse, friend or other relative as the greatest source of help (described earlier in this chapter). For patients in stoma care districts the stoma care nurse figures prominently. Few patients mentioned the district nurse (Wade 1989). (See also Table 15.1 in the next chapter.)

Apart from the referral to the appropriate agency on discharge, patients also need to know how to order a supply of appliances and should be given a sufficient supply to go home with to last them until their own supplies are obtained (discussed more fully in Ch. 16). A contact number for the stoma care nurse is given, as well as written information on changing the appliance which helps to allay patients' fears that they may have forgotten everything by the time they reach home. Useful leaflets come from the World Council of Enterostomal Therapists (WCET), and one for each type of stoma is available (see Appendix). Just having something written down can aid patients' transition to the community situation and take away a few of the worries. Information is also given to the patient's GP (Fig. 14.3).

The most important role of the stoma care nurse is the maintenance of contact with patients and their families after discharge – to be a resource, to reassure when changes happen, but gradually, during the rehabilitation period, to aid the patient to a recovery that enables him or her to lead a normal and productive life within the community.

STOMA CARE REQUIREMENTS

Dear Doctor
Your patient was
discharged on

HOSPITAL _____

ADDRESS _____

_____

To be retained by
G.P.

Date _____

And his/her current
stoma care
requirements are
set out below

Your nearest stoma care nurse is: _____

_____

Telephone Number _____

Patient's Name

SURNAME (Mr/Mrs/Miss) _____

FORENAMES _____

ADDRESS _____

G.P.'s Name

DR _____

ADDRESS _____

_____

APPLIANCE	BRAND	SIZE	CODE SERIES No.	NUMBER IN UNIT PACK	APPROX No. REQUIRED IN 4 WEEKS
Pouch Closed					
Pouch Drainable					
Flange					
Pouch Closure					
Other					

Figure 14.3 Discharge: informing the GP

15

Community care

COMMUNITY CARE TODAY

Successfully rehabilitating the stoma patient in the community means continuing the care provided by the hospital and preparing the patient for a new phase of life (Black 1990). In a study by Pringle et al (1997) it was suggested that the poor quality of life and the feelings of stigma experienced by many stoma patients appear to be affected by the level of support that is available to them once they are discharged from hospital. It seems that the passage from hospital to home has always been seen as a weak link in the chain of continuing care and support for the new stoma patient (Rubin & Devlin 1987).

In some areas the stoma care nurse from the hospital continues the care in the home situation until the patient is rehabilitated. In other areas the hospital stoma care nurse, in liaison with the ward staff, will discharge the patient to the community stoma care nurse, who will then arrange to visit the patient and make a detailed assessment of the patient and his or her needs. Sometimes there will not be a stoma care nurse, either in hospital or in the community, and the patient is referred to the district nurse for assessment, supervision and general help and support in the management of the stoma.

Successful rehabilitation of the stoma patient in the community depends on several factors:

1. Understanding the type of stoma constructed and whether it is temporary or permanent
2. Understanding which type of appliance is the correct one to use

3. Having a knowledge of alternative appliances if the original is found to be difficult to use or causing skin problems
4. Trouble-shooting for common problems sometimes seen after stoma surgery (Black 1997a).

The stoma care nurse who works across both the hospital and the community is ideally placed to help with the isolation that the patient feels on first being at home. The stoma care nurse acts as a coordinator between the family and patient and other agencies such as the GP, social services, district nurse, Macmillan nurse, other specialist nurses and the health visitor if an infant with a stoma is involved. Patients and their families or carers expect the stoma care nurse to provide guidance in management issues and provide a credible authority in the management of patients and their rehabilitation (Righter 1995).

The skills that the patient has learned in hospital will often have to be adapted in the home situation and relearned. With the worry of discharge much of the practical management of stoma care is often forgotten or becomes unsure and the patient loses the help that has hitherto been available 24 hours a day. The cold, stark reality of learning to live with a stoma begins to be felt.

For some patients discharged home the outcome is going to be poor. They may have colorectal cancer, which may be considerably advanced, and have to start adjuvant therapy in a few weeks. For a minority there will be no adjuvant therapy as the disease has progressed too far and the patient and his or her family will be coming to terms with a stoma and progressive disease from which the patient will shortly die. The role for the stoma care nurse in this situation is to maintain the therapeutic relationship, to support the family, who need to express their emotions, and also support and encourage the patient, however dismal the outcome will be (Pringle et al 1997).

Wade (1989), in her study of stoma care nurses and their patients, looked at the formal support a stoma patient receives on discharge from hospital (see also Table 15.1). In districts where there were stoma care nurses, 93% of patients had received at least one visit up to 10 weeks

after surgery. Only 7% of patients in non stoma care nurse districts had seen or made contact with a stoma care nurse, who was often a stoma care nurse their relatives knew and contacted, or whom the patient had met informally elsewhere. Some district nurses had asked the specialist nurse to visit patients with difficult problems. In many areas where there was a stoma care nurse covering either hospital and community or community, the initial postoperative visit was within 48 hours of discharge. If the specialist nurse could not visit at an early date, the district nurse was asked to call on the patient within the first 48 hours. (See Table 15.1.)

The full impact of the consequences of stoma surgery is often not felt until patients return home and realise that they now have to cope on their own, with only occasional visits by either the stoma care nurse or the district nurse. Even though they know that the nurse is just a telephone call away, many patients feel that they should not bother the nurse, who is always so busy.

The only ongoing contact some stoma patients have is with the GP, who may have little knowledge of or time to deal with the practical and psychological problems that stoma patients encounter. If there is a stoma care nurse in the community, he or she will be the person with the necessary knowledge and skills to advise, if necessary, the GP. Wade (1989) suggests that it is part of the stoma care nurse's role to assess the living conditions of the patient, to provide the continued support necessary to increase the patient's confidence and self-esteem and to mobilise other resources where needed, liaising and coordinating with other appropriate agencies as necessary. Without doubt, care of the stoma patient in the community by a nurse speeds the patient's rehabilitation and return to a normal and productive life. Regular visits to patients' homes can establish a rapport with patients and their families, and the nurse may be treated as a confidante, to whom the patient can turn when there are problems with the stoma.

Home visits to stoma care patients enable the nurse to view the patient from a holistic angle and to assess any real or potential problem areas that may occur. They also give the nurse a chance

Table 15.1 Patients' perceptions of who has been of most help since discharge (from Wade 1989)

Areas	Stoma care nurse n=176 %	Non stoma care nurse n=87 %	All n=263 %
Spouse	40.9	46.6	43.0
Other relatives	17.6	15.9	17.1
Friends/neighbours	4.0	6.8	4.9
Stoma nurse	19.9	0.0	13.3
Company nurse	1.1	8.0	3.4
District nurse	1.1	11.5	4.6
GP	2.3	4.5	3.0
Social services	2.3	0.0	1.5
Patient	2.8	2.3	2.7
Other	2.3	1.1	1.6
No one particularly	5.7	3.4	4.9
Total	100.0	100.1	100.0

to meet any other members of the family who will play a role in caring for the stoma patient and help in their rehabilitation. If carers have problems about the care of the patient, they will often broach these with the stoma care nurse during home visits, possibly taking the nurse to one side, or beginning a conversation at the garden gate or in another room to voice their current concerns about the patient. Patients should at no time be made to feel that they are being talked about behind their backs, or that their diagnosis or prognosis is being discussed without them. If there is not a suitable room or other area that the nurse and carer can discreetly withdraw to, the nurse should suggest that the carer perhaps telephones or comes to the clinic where the carer can quietly discuss any worries or concerns. Often carers do not feel that the patient is telling them everything and think that something is being held back. This may be quite irrational, but it is not unexpected where patients and their families have been given a bad prognosis. In cases where the patient will need palliative care, which may be initiated at home and continued there, there is often the fear of the patient dying at home. Carers may be worried that they will not know what to do, who to call and how they will cope. However, some patients and their families will have adjusted to impending death at home and are prepared. Where there are fears, they must be addressed by the stoma care nurse and support and reassurance given.

A major part of the stoma care nurse's home visit is to assess the bathroom facilities and how the patient can adapt the facilities to his or her needs for stoma care management. Changes may be needed in the bathroom, such as bath rails, shower facilities, or a bath board to allow strip showers for patients unable to immerse themselves fully in the bath. Many district nurses and stoma care nurses work in areas that have poor housing stock, including houses without bathroom facilities, without hot water, and even some still without electricity and with only an outside toilet. Nurses who do not work in the community are often surprised at how and where people live, having expected their patients to be living in accommodation similar to their own. However, it must be said that nurses who regularly work in the community are not often taken by surprise. The hospital nurse who is perhaps spending the day out with the stoma care nurse in the community may be taken aback to find patients living in canal boats, on fair ground traveller sites, on a gypsy encampment, in prison, under plastic tarpaulin next to a motorway with a shotgun next to them, in bed and breakfast accommodation, or in accommodation for the homeless with six people in one room and 20 plus sharing a single toilet. Outbreaks of shigella dysentery are common in such conditions and very dangerous for the patient with an ileostomy. It is suggested that life with a stoma demands adaptation and changes to ingrained habits of personal hygiene, but if the facilities are not there or likely to be there, the nurse must help the patient adapt to what is available. Nurses should also remember that some patients are illiterate and may not have disclosed this to anyone before. To reinforce teaching with written material may not be appropriate in this situation and innovation will be needed. Taped information on caring for a colostomy, ileostomy and urostomy is available from one of the major ostomy companies, but a tape recorder is needed and also electricity to plug it into. If this does not meet requirements, instructions for organising care can be done in picture mode. Pictures of each part of the procedure – cut from the teaching booklets, computerised graphics, or drawn – can be heat-sealed to give a protective and washable surface and the sheet will remain sturdy for a considerable time.

Many stoma care nurses offer an open facility clinic either in the community or in the hospital. Patients may access these clinics whenever they have a problem, or in the hospital situation may take the advantage of the clinic while visiting other clinics or other areas of the hospital. The aim of a stoma clinic (in the hospital or in the community) is to fulfil the needs of that particular group and it can be done in a number of ways. The clinic can:

- Prepare and counsel the patient preoperatively and support the family or carer
- Be a resource where any potential stoma problems can be identified and corrected
- Provide information on current surgical techniques in stoma surgery and discuss issues not only with stoma patients and their families, but also with members of the medical team who require information and help
- Hold samples of a range of appliances to suit all needs and eventualities, so that a patient who has a problem with an appliance can consider other types of appliances.

Open access nurse led clinics allow the patient to retain the locus of control and they are not regimented into the biomedical model.

Stoma care in the community at present remains fragmented and diverse and without a common goal. Yet a study by Jefferies (1993) suggested that where patients are assured of support within both the hospital and community, and where this support is forthcoming, patients will feel better able to cope and adjust to living with a stoma.

INTEGRATED CARE PATHWAYS

In the ideal world there would be an integrated approach to the care of the stoma patient with both professional and voluntary helpers, such as those from the stoma care associations, helping the new stoma patient through the process of rehabilitation. Stringer (1985) suggests that there will be no substantial decline in patients with a stoma in the next decade, and that the need for stoma care will remain as acute as it was when the then Department of Health and Social Services published the blueprint for stoma care in the UK (DHSS 1978), which outlined the need for:

- Psychological preparation of the patient and relatives before surgery, when this is possible
- A suitably sited stoma and provision of an acceptable and well-fitting appliance
- Advice on skin care and stoma management
- Psychological support postoperatively with problems that may arise
- Continued care and advice after discharge from hospital.

Responsibility to the patient before and after surgery lies with surgeon and GP, with specialist care in coping with the adaptation and attitudinal change given by the stoma therapist, or if not available, the district nurse. In attempting to give a smooth transition from hospital to home, integrated care pathways organise and deliver true multidisciplinary, evidence based care which is appropriate for an individual.

Managing health care effectively depends on close monitoring of the patient and the family needs throughout the period in which care is needed. Multidisciplinary care programmes are tailored to suit the needs of an individual and allow for better planned patient care, higher service quality and a smoother patient care process. Wilson (1996) states:

Integrated care management views the multidisciplinary approaches to collaborating care delivery by activity, cost, and quality; and uses a process approach to problem and outcome based care delivery. Involving patients and their carers in determining the process and outcomes of care provides a route to better communication, patient and staff satisfaction and the overall quality of care.

In using a pathway as a staged plan, Wilson (1996) notes the appropriate use and timing of procedures in relation to patient recovery. The interdisciplinary approach helps to reduce clinical variation in clinical practice across the different care settings, while continuing to maintain quality patient care.

The Department of Health document EL (93) 115, entitled *Improving clinical effectiveness*, (Department of Health 1993), outlines clearly the need for the multidisciplinary team to identify and develop evidence based clinical guidelines and protocols of care. Integrating and designing the services around the specific needs of patients helps to reduce patient uncertainty and delays and empowers patients to become partners in their own care. It eliminates duplication and unexplained variations in clinical practice between the multidisciplinary team members and is able to carry out interdisciplinary audit through goals, outcomes and variance tracking, thereby improving the patient's quality of care.

To achieve successful care paths there has to be top down commitment and ownership from the bottom, and the care path framework needs to be agreed from existing records. In developing the care path, all team members need to be involved in small working groups. Selecting and writing care paths in multidisciplinary teams helps to define ownership and communication. The teams review, change and update the pathway and this effective teamwork promotes better communication between the professionals and the patient. Integrated care pathways support the hospital consultant and the general practitioner, enabling them to work together to provide care to bridge the traditional divide between hospital and community care. True integrated care path-

ways work across both the hospital and the community setting, with a pathway of care existing for an individual with a particular disease. They also offer the community practitioners a framework to work within to help prevent the possibility of mismanagement. Therefore integrated care pathways should effectively reduce the need for repeated admission to hospital and enable patients to contribute to all aspects of the provision of services, from assessment of need through to evaluation of the delivered service. This empowers patients and encourages them to assume an appropriate level of responsibility for helping shape the services they receive.

Consistency of practice is important in all health care settings. In many areas care is recorded up to eight times in various professional records and communication between those involved in care can be haphazard and inefficient. To improve the quality of the clinical process, reduce risk and control costs it is essential to eliminate inappropriate variations and documentation. Research into health care both in the UK and America shows that it is the process rather than the people that makes a system break down (Berwick 1989). Pathways are therefore ideally situated to improve the integrated care process which is the key to increased quality of care for the patient.

POSSIBLE COMPLICATIONS IN THE COMMUNITY CARE SETTING

Stomal complications

Patients with a stoma face a variety of special stresses which include possible social isolation, low self-esteem, conflicts over body image and a sense of powerlessness and incompetence. Such stresses affect their psychological well-being, and their reaction may be withdrawal from the family, work and group activities. The surgeon who considers a stoma to be necessary as a curative or palliative procedure may focus on the technical aspects of the operation, rather than the social and emotional impact of a stoma. While providing support for the stoma patient, the nurse will encounter problems and complications which can occur as a result of the surgery.

The complications associated with a stoma may be categorised as those that require surgical or medical treatment (stenosis, prolapse, paralytic ileus and parastomal hernias) and those that can be attended to by the nurse (skin problems, leakage, diarrhoea and rejection of the stoma).

Skin problems (Box 15.1)

Adaptation to life with a stoma depends to a large extent on the health of the peristomal skin. This area of skin can become damaged in various ways, and the resulting discomfort or pain can make the use of an appliance difficult. Skin problems are the major complications facing the stoma care nurse or district nurse.

When a patient has stoma surgery, whether elective or emergency, the skin is usually healthy. After a few days, or after some time at home, some patients develop a skin problem. The stoma patient may have a minor skin problem at first but think little of it, or think that it is not worth bothering the stoma care nurse about, but gradually the skin deteriorates to the point where the patient finds it too painful to put on an appliance, or the appliances continue to leak, so perpetuating the problem. Most stoma patients have few if any skin problems, but for those who do it is an added stressor.

The skin provides protection against physical and chemical agents and against bacterial invasion. This protection depends on an intact epidermis. When the epidermis is damaged by infection, by constant exposure to moisture, or by stripping of adhesive material from the skin, the protective action of the skin is compromised. Excessive washing of the skin, as is practised by some patients, removes all its protective oils and reduces its water repellent properties. Often though, through misguided information, patients are told not to use soap on the peristomal skin area. It is important that when an appliance is changed the skin is washed in the normal way, as after a bowel evacuation. Water alone cannot remove faecal enzymes. These remain on the skin, especially those from ileostomy output, and if the skin is not cleansed properly and thoroughly, skin problems may arise. The normal soap that the family uses is perfectly satisfactory for this purpose (Black 1998b). It is essential to determine the cause of a skin problem. The nurse must therefore spend time with the patient to determine the cause and to ensure that the patient knows how to take care of the peristomal skin, and that the appliance fits snugly, is easy to apply and to remove, and is non allergenic. The nurse needs to review the patient's diet and to look for any underlying skin problems. Removal and correction of an underlying problem will often allow the patient to be able to continue with the original appliance, but if the patient has to change to a different appliance this can be an added stressor.

Some patients may have to undergo radiotherapy and chemotherapy after stoma surgery and these treatments may cause problems with the skin. With both treatments diarrhoea may occur and the patient can feel quite debilitated. Often, during treatment such as this the use of a two-piece appliance may be beneficial as the flange may be left in situ for several days, but enables the appliance to be changed as often as necessary (Black 1989b).

Occasionally hypersensitivity to either the plastic, the appliance or the adhesive may occur. A total change may relieve the situation, but it may be necessary to patch test the patient with all the possible appliances and adhesives to find the one least irritating to the patient's skin. It is quite rare to have a patient who cannot tolerate any of today's adhesives on the skin. In trials it was shown that Stomahesive® had a significantly less irritating effect on the skin when removed daily or weekly, and concluded that it was the nature of the adhesive that was important and not the frequency of removal (Marks et al 1978).

A few patients develop allergic dermatitis after using adhesives and plastics to which they had no previous reaction. Dermatitis may either be allergic or due to direct irritants. Skin cleansers and materials used for the preparation of the peristomal skin may cause reactions. Some patients feel that disinfectant is required to clean the stoma but this must be discouraged by the nurse. Due to weight change or poor siting of the stoma, faecal and urinary matter can track along gullies in the skin. This can cause the skin to become sore and an irritant dermatitis may develop. The gullies can be filled with paste to make the area flush before applying the flange or bag, so preventing tracking of faecal or urinary output onto other skin.

Other skin problems include eczema, which commonly affects damp areas of the body such as under the flange, especially in warmer weather when the patient is likely to perspire more. Psoriatic lesions may develop in the operation scar if the patient has psoriasis and may make application of a bag difficult if it develops around the stoma.

One of the unpleasant skin manifestations of inflammatory bowel disease – both Crohn's and ulcerative colitis – is pyoderma gangrenosum. In some patients, pyoderma that is present pre-operatively will resolve once the bowel disease improves, but for others it does not. Local treatment of pyoderma is not often helpful, although local irrigation with calcium hypochlorite can ease the irritation. Antibiotics do not have much effect and corticosteroids are often necessary. In some patients the disease can be particularly resistant and higher doses of steroids may be necessary. Immunosupressive therapy may be useful in resistant cases.

Infection of the peristomal skin may be caused by either bacteria or fungi. Bacterial infection of the peristomal skin, commonly caused by staphylococci or coliforms, may require systemic antibiotic therapy. However, it must be remembered that systemic antibiotics can promote fungal infections such as candida. The use of a topical cream or ointment containing a steroid, antifungal and antibacterial may be more appropriate in clearing a local infection.

Trauma in the epidermis can be caused by too frequent changing of an appliance, particularly if a one-piece system is used. Stoma patients should be advised to change the appliance only when necessary in order to prevent repeated damage to the epidermis. It may be necessary to change from a one-piece to two-piece appliance to avoid unnecessary bag changes.

As noted above, radiotherapy to the abdominal area causes the skin to become reddened and tender. When this occurs, the patient may have trouble in using an appliance. There is an added problem of radiotherapy causing diarrhoea and looseness of faeces, and this can further aggravate the skin.

Skin changes occur with age, stress and illness. These cause a change in the permeability of the skin, and patients who have used a stoma appliance with no problems for some time may suddenly find themselves with an appliance that does not adhere and starts to leak or has to be changed frequently. It may be possible to correct the underlying cause so that the patient may continue to use the appliance that he or she is familiar with. However, for some patients it may be necessary to change the appliance totally and such a change is often difficult for an elderly patient to accept. A full explanation for the change should be given sensitively.

Skin problems in urostomy patients are caused by the contact of urine with the peristomal skin. If the peristomal skin becomes red and sore, a suitable barrier cream for peristomal skin should be applied after careful washing and drying of the skin. Phosphate crystals can form on the peristomal skin and stoma. These crystals can be removed by dabbing half-strength acetic acid (household vinegar) on the affected area for several days when the appliance is changed. The patient should also be encouraged to drink more fluid. When the urine is alkaline, there may be bluish discoloration of the peristomal skin and the appliance. This can be rectified by acidifying the urine with ascorbic acid (vitamin C) and increasing the patient's fluid intake.

Hyperplasia of the epidermis, which presents as a thickening of the skin in the peristomal area, results from continual exposure of the skin to urine. This can be prevented by ensuring the appliance fits snugly around the stoma. Candida infections are prone to occur in moist, warm, covered areas and tend to be a common problem with urostomies. An anticandidal cream or powder will combat the infection and assist adherence of the appliance.

Folliculitis is caused by tearing a hair follicle. In patients who are particularly hairy, it is advisable to shave the peristomal area with an electric razor

---

Box 15.1 Possible causes of skin irritation

Faecal leakage
Ill-fitting appliance
Poorly sited stoma
Scars close to the stoma
Complicated stoma

Mechanical irritation
Adhesive
Kinking of adhesive material
Measures used to clean skin
Substances used to clean skin

Allergy/hypersensitivity
Any substance that comes into contact with the
peristomal skin
Substances used to clean skin
Skin preparations

Sweating
Fungal
Bacterial

Pre-existing skin disease
Eczema
Psoriasis
Pyoderma

---

before the application of the bag or flange. If a wet razor is used, care must be taken not to cut the stoma. Folliculitis can be treated topically.

Other stomal problems

Hernias. Peristomal hernias (see Plate 10) occur in about 20% of patients who have a stoma raised. They are caused by a weakness of the abdominal muscle through which the stoma passes. Ideally the stoma should be sited in the abdominus rectus sheath which helps to protect the stoma and prevent herniation. Unless the herniation is strangulated or causing severe restriction to the quality of life of the patient, surgical correction is unlikely. It is often difficult to correct a hernia in this area and may involve resiting of the stoma and extensive surgery, only to find that it happens again. Help with herniation can be given by ordering for a patient a girdle to support the hernia. A hole is left in the girdle for the appliance to come through to allow emptying as necessary. A hole much larger than 60 cm will make the girdle ineffective, as most of the hernia will protrude through it and be unsupported.

The stoma care nurse or district nurse can refer the patient to the local hospital appliance department where, if they have an orthotist, the patient can go to be measured for a support belt or girdle. Many patients, by virtue of their age or disability, are unable to go to the hospital and the nurse can arrange for a domiciliary visit from one of the appliance contractors in the ostomy industry. In order to give maximum support, the belt should be put on first thing on waking, before the hernia starts to protrude.

Prolapse. Prolapse of the stoma (see Plate 11) can be very alarming for the patient and can occur without any apparent reason. Prolapse is seen more frequently in patients who have a temporary transverse colostomy and occurs in about 20% of these patients. The prolapse can extend significantly and look offensive and frightening to the patient, as well as causing appliance problems and leakage. A suitable larger appliance should be used with an adequate sized aperture to exclude damage to the stoma. The only solution to this problem is to close the temporary stoma as soon as possible, but almost invariably the patient with this type of stoma is too ill and it falls to the community nurse or stoma care nurse to cope with the problem. Patients are often sent by the GP to the A&E department when a prolapse is seen. The prolapse is reduced with ice wrapped in a towel and applied over the stoma. When the oedema has subsided the prolapse is manipulated back through the abdominal wall. If available, a rigid plastic shield is applied over the stoma bag and kept in place with a belt to try and contain the prolapse (Black 1998b).

Paralytic ileus. Paralytic ileus, though relatively uncommon after stoma surgery, may be caused by trauma, either by accidents or by excessive manipulation of the gut during surgery.

Retraction. Retraction of the stoma may occur if the bowel is brought to the abdominal surface under tension and too little bowel is mobilised during fashioning of the stoma. It can also occur if there is inadequate fixation of the stoma to the abdominal surface, and postoperatively if the patient gains a lot of weight.

Stenosis. This can be caused by the formation of scar tissue, particularly if the stoma becomes necrotic due to infection around the stoma with separation of the bowel and skin. Often it is not advisable or suitable for the patient to have surgery to refashion the stoma and the stoma care nurse or community nurse will be advised to help the patient regularly dilate the stoma to keep it patent. This can be done once or twice a day with a gloved, lubricated finger, starting with a small finger and moving to the next. Alternatively a set of metal dilators can be used (such as Hegar's or St Mark's), again starting with the smallest, moving on to a larger size. If dilation keeps the stoma patent, surgery can be avoided.

Stress. Time spent reducing stress is time well spent. There are inevitable stresses living with a stoma and the stoma care nurse and community nurse, armed with the necessary knowledge, are in the ideal place to help relieve and rectify these problems. Once they are reassured that there is nothing untoward happening and that life can carry on, patients should be able to continue their normal lifestyle.

16

Prescribing in the community

SUPPLIES OF STOMA GOODS

When stoma patients are ready to leave hospital and return home, one of their biggest anxieties is how and where they will be able to obtain appliances. Either on the day of discharge or the day before, the patient will have been visited on the ward by the stoma care nurse who will advise on obtaining appliances, either at a local pharmacy or through a delivery service. A prescription will have to be obtained from the GP regardless of which service the patient uses. If the patient is under 60 years of age and the stoma is permanent, an exemption certificate is obtained by filling in a form obtainable from the stoma care nurse, GP's surgery or post office. The form is filled in by the patient, taken to the GP and signed, and sent off to the Family Health Services Association (FHSA), and in time the exemption certificate duly arrives. Patients who have a temporary stoma are, if possible, given enough supplies by the hospital to last until their return for reversal of the stoma. If this is not possible, patients will be expected to pay for their prescriptions at the usual rate. Since 1 April 1999 patients who hold an exemption certificate have been expected to show it when going to the pharmacy to order their supplies. Patients, both male and female, over the age of 60 are eligible for free prescriptions.

What are the advantages and disadvantages of using a pharmacy or a delivery service? When discharge from hospital is near, patients should be told how their supplies are obtained. They should be told that the local pharmacy will supply appliances, but that the pharmacy does not keep them on the shelf and they have to be ordered in. Alternatively, the supplies may be delivered and the nurse will advise on a delivery service. There are many excellent delivery services available to the stoma care nurse and all deliver to the home within 24 hours of the order being placed. Delivery is discreet, personal and free. Many patients are keen to use their local pharmacy as they have been obtaining their drugs and other goods there for many years and often the pharmacist is a friend who can help and advise. In recent years there has been input from the National Pharmaceutical Association (NPA) to local pharmacies who belong to the organisation to do more for stoma patients, not just hand the supplies over the counter. Many pharmacies have seen a decline in numbers of stoma patients using their services as patients have changed to delivery services recommended by the stoma care nurse or seen by the patient at stoma care open days. Patients sometimes change to a delivery service, having started with the pharmacy, because they are given disposable bags and cleaning wipes free, as part of the delivery service. All delivery services endeavour to have a 24-hour service, provided that the appliances required are in stock. If only one box is available, it will usually be immediately dispatched to the patient, with the rest following very soon afterwards. Delivery services are able to cut appliances for patients, which is especially helpful if the stoma is an awkward shape that does not conform to the factory pre-cut round holes. For an appliance to be cut, a template of the stoma size and shape needs to be sent. When local pharmacies saw what patients could be offered with a delivery service, with the help of the NPA many felt they could offer wipes and disposable bags, and a few will even cut stoma appliances for their customers. Some local pharmacies will deliver goods for patients who cannot easily go to the shop and this can be a great help for the elderly as the supplies can be bulky and difficult to carry. Delivery services are not only useful for patients in rural areas or on isolated islands in the UK. Many people in cities and towns find a delivery service useful

as, after undergoing major stoma surgery, they are unable to go out for a long time. Such patients may have no family members able to collect their supplies for them, and there may be little or no input from social services if the patient does not fall into the right criteria; without home delivery these patients would not be able to obtain supplies. The first home visit of the stoma care nurse enables the nurse to enquire if the patient has received supplies, whether from the pharmacy or delivery service, and it is best if this first visit can take place within 48 hours after discharge from hospital, especially if there has been a hold-up in the patient receiving supplies. Patients should be encouraged to order a new supply when they start the last box of an order to give time for the supplies to come. When ordering through a pharmacy it may take up to 5 days from placement of the order to the arrival of the supplies at the pharmacy. If the order is left until there are only three or four bags left, patients may run out of bags while awaiting the arrival of the order. When approaching long public holiday periods such as Christmas, it is wise to order early (say in November) as there is often a rush on wholesalers for supplies.

THE COST OF STOMA MANAGEMENT

Costs

The cost of caring for the stoma patient in the community takes a large part of the GP's budget and many GPs are now querying this cost, especially as stoma goods are low volume, high priced goods. From April 1999, general practices in England will become members of primary care groups (PCGs) and they will have unified budgets for prescribing hospital and community health services, therefore it is vital that prescribing costs are kept under control. Stoma care and its products is an area of prescribing that the majority of GPs find difficult to assess and in which they rely on the stoma care nurse for prescribing details and information. If a patient came to a GP and asked for stoma bags it is likely that the GP would not be able to prescribe the correct appliance or aperture size for the patient, unless the patient provides information on the appliance currently being used. If the appliance is not on the GP's current database, the doctor may think that the appliance is not available. Looking through the drug tariff (part ix C), however, shows that there is a myriad of stoma appliances to choose from.

In 1997 stoma goods accounted for 1.3 million prescription items costing £89 000 000 – 2% of prescribing costs for England in that year. Stoma goods, after the first prescription, are provided on a repeat request basis and repeat prescriptions are usually signed without question, as most GPs have little knowledge of the products. Only in the face of escalating costs do they frantically search for areas that can be cut back on and fall upon stoma care, seeing it as low volume, high priced turnover.

AUDITING STOMA PRESCRIBING

Some accessory products may have been recommended by the stoma care nurse for the GP to prescribe as a one time only prescription, but unless the product is removed from the patient's prescription record it can go on being prescribed at each request. For GPs the use of prescribing analysis and cost data (PACT) can be a useful tool to audit stoma prescribing within the PCG. Prescribing information is collated and kept by the Prescribing Prescription Authority (PPA) and includes the name, cost and number of items dispensed. This information is put onto a database. Specific information by categories defined by the British National Formulary (BNF) is made available at national, health authority and practice levels. Rates and costs of prescribing are analysed, together with other comparative information. PACT includes information on prescribing costs, number of items prescribed and generic prescribing. PACT information allows examination of a specific therapeutic area such as stoma care and, along with consultation with the stoma care nurse, practice formularies for stoma appliances and accessories can be drawn up. Besides the formulary of products, the GP and stoma care nurse can draw up a protocol of what the nurse

is able to offer potential patients who are about to undergo stoma surgery and what may be offered to the patient who has had stoma surgery. In close working with the practice and the GP, the stoma care nurse can provide a service that entails:

- Preoperative counselling for patients in their own homes or the surgery, with family members
- Continuing care at home postoperatively, through rehabilitation and back to work, if appropriate
- Support and education of family and/or carer
- Rationalisation and impartial advice with regard to stoma appliances
- Liaison with all members of the primary care team
- Help and advice on any stomal problems that may occur
- Close control on expenditure on stoma appliances
- Yearly audit of practice stoma patients
- Introduction of new appliances and update of practice computer
- Educational programmes for all practice staff.

Majeed (1998) suggests that many general practitioners may not have the expertise to identify inappropriate or excessive usage of certain products. Hence the next stage in assessing stoma care product prescribing is discussion on the range of products with the specialist stoma care nurse. Some areas that should be examined are:

- Is the balance between the use of one-piece and two-piece appliances correct?
- Are patients with two-piece appliances being prescribed the correct ratio of flanges to bags?
- Are accessories being used appropriately?
- Who funds the stoma care nurse? (This will be discussed further in Ch. 25, on the role of the specialist nurse.)

It is estimated that the current number of stoma patients living in the UK is between 80 000 and 100 000 and the general trend is static/slightly decreasing (see Box 16.1).

It appears that GPs find the large and constantly changing number of stoma products

Box 16.1	Patient numbers		
Permanent colostomy		39 000	39.8%
Permanent ileostomy		34 600	34.6%
Permanent urostomy		22 500	22.5%
Temporary stoma		3100	3.1%
New patients (approximately 20 000 per annum)			
Permanent colostomy		6800	34.3%
Permanent ileostomy		2280	11.4%
Permanent urostomy		1980	9.9%
Temporary stoma		8860	44.3%

that become available bewildering. It is estimated that the costs of colostomy, ileostomy, urostomy and two-piece systems accounts for 90% of stoma care spending and it is suggested that practices that spend more than 10% of their total costs on other products in this area should examine their spending and determine if there is scope for rationalisation (Majeed 1998). This can be done by an audit of the stoma patients and the appliances and accessories used.

The audit cycle

Audit is an emotive word in the world of health care today. For many it is a threatening exercise, with the possibility of showing discrepancies or lack of quality care. For those who embrace it, audit enables health care practitioners to redefine practice and offer better care, and allows identification of areas where money can be saved. The medical definition of audit is, 'the systematic, critical analysis of the quality of care, including the procedures used for diagnosis and treatment, the use of resources, and the resulting outcome and quality of life for the patient.' The purpose of audit is to identify opportunities and implement improvements in the following three areas:

1. Quality of medical care
2. Training and continuing education
3. Effective use of resources.

Auditing can promote excellence, aid education and improve patient outcomes. It can also help provide a more structured and formal setting for agreeing standards by which to practice. This can help minimise national variations. As such,

audit is a method of evaluating healthcare and involves:

- Observing and discussing practice to find out what actually happens
- Setting a standard of practice and so defining what ought to happen
- Comparing observed practice with the standard
- Implementing change
- Observing practice after changes have been implemented.

These five activities constitute the audit cycle. For an audit to be successful, there must be feedback of information, and it must include mechanisms for implementing change if problems have been identified. Common topics for audit are the structure and use of resources, accessibility of resources, communications and outcomes of care relating to social, medical and economic terms (Black 1998a). In auditing practice and evolving standards for stoma patients and GPs, self-selected criteria would involve the way patient stoma problems are addressed, coping with complications of the stoma, advice to help the patient live with a stoma, and appliance usage and optimums. Audit data which can demonstrate a reduction in certain measurable costs (the number of prescriptions issued and quantity of appliances supplied) can only be of value to the National Health Service as a whole and is to be encouraged.

Demonstrating the value of audit

In demonstrating how an audit within PCGs can be of value, an audit of stoma care prescribing using PACT data was taken across twelve practices. The data was analysed to show:

- The total quantity and cost of appliances and accessories prescribed
- Quantity and cost of appliances by stoma type
- Choice of appliance by manufacturer
- Selection of one-piece versus two-piece.

The stoma care nursing input within these areas was provided by NHS stoma care nurses, sponsored stoma care nurses and company stoma care nurses. The audit aimed to identify potential areas for cost savings, and also whether there were any differences in stoma care prescribing costs where the stoma care nursing was not wholly NHS, and whether the prescribing practice of stoma appliances and accessories favoured the range offered by the nurse's sponsoring company in the non NHS areas.

It appeared that few of the practices could supply accurate data of true stoma patient numbers for the audit period, so an estimation of the number of patients was made on the quantity of appliances used, based on an optimum of needs:

- Colostomy – two bags per day
- Ileostomy – one bag per day
- Urostomy – one bag per day.

Estimated numbers of stoma patients were:

- Colostomy – 118.3
- Ileostomy – 73.3
- Urostomy – 12.5.

The total number of patients on the combined practices list was 161 600, and the cost of stoma care to these practices over the financial year April 1995 to March 1996 was £287 535. The highest cost per treated patient was £1803 in a company stoma care nurse area with a high usage of accessories. The lowest cost was £1144 in an area with a sponsored nurse, mainly because of high two-piece usage and low accessory usage. In asking if the balance of use between one-piece and two-piece appliances is correct within the prescribing of a GP's practice, Majeed (1998) suggests that the potential to reuse a flange on a two-piece appliance gives a potentially cheaper appliance than a one-piece system. However, stoma care nurses have said that they find it easier to start a patient on a one-piece system as it is easier to teach its use to the patient in view of the short time patients now spend in hospital. In addition, many patients prefer a one-piece system and consumer preference must be taken into account. Comparison of the practices' expenditure demonstrated the significant differences in the mix of products and appliances prescribed, with accessories such as skin products, deodorants and bag covers accounting for as little as 6.9% or as much as 35.7% of expenditure. As previously mentioned, any practice which spends significantly more than 10% of total costs on other products in this area should examine their prescribing to determine if there is scope for rationalisation.

The average cost for each treated colostomy patient was £1377. The lowest was £1076 where predominantly two-piece colostomy systems were used. It was noted that the higher usage of two-piece colostomy appliances gave the practice a lower cost per treated patient.

The average cost per ileostomy patient was £794, but in one practice where more two-piece appliances were used the cost was lower than average, equalling £760.

Because of the smaller number of urostomy patients, appliance usage tended to be exclusively one-piece or two-piece. The average cost was £1365, but the choice of a cheaper one-piece appliance brought the cost down to £1054.

In areas where there were company or sponsored nurses, the range of appliances prescribed was far smaller and frequently favoured the sponsoring company. Even with a dominant market two-piece supplier, the audit showed that there was evidence that sponsorship did influence the choice of appliances prescribed.

Audit conclusion

If all patients in the audited practices who were using one-piece appliances were changed to two-piece appliances it is estimated that £46 000 could be saved across these practices (an estimated 16% of total expenditure). There might also be a reduced need for accessory products. The highest proportion of accessory products and one-piece appliances was in a company nurse area. In 7 out of 10 areas accessories accounted for 5–10% of practice expenditure. Table 16.1 shows the annual savings that could be made in the above audit.

Wade (1989) suggested that more than one in 10 stoma patients had difficulty in establishing their equipment supply, with more than half the sample having to go to their GP just for a prescription for stoma appliances. The necessity to place an order in advance often meant that the

Table 16.1   Estimate of annual savings per patient when two-piece appliances are used

Stoma type	One-piece	Two-piece	Saving
Colostomy	£1380	£1040	£340
Ileostomy	£780	£726	£54
Urostomy	£1575	£1263	£312

patient had to make two visits to the chemist. In 1989, when Wade interviewed her patient sample, delivery services such as we have now were not available. She suggested that a lot of problems for the new stoma patient could be avoided if the stoma care nurse was allowed to prescribe. This reality is now approaching, and in 1998 the government announced that nurse prescribing would be rolled out nationally and that £14 million was being allocated to it. It had initially been thought that nurse prescribing was in danger of being lost in the changes in the health service and in community care. The roll out is still on schedule and implementation guidance has been given to health authorities from the NHS Executive. There will be a national programme for training all eligible practitioners and community nurses will be able to access courses over the next 3 years (until March 2001). The Association for Nurse Prescribing has a handbook which has information on prescribing issues and a directory of useful information and references.

17

Patient organisations

Self-help groups in ostomy care have evolved since the 1930s to help the patient who has undergone a surgical operation to form a stoma. A common assumption is that mutual aid groups exist to help both helper and helpee. Reissman (1965) described the helper therapy principle, implying that it is the helper who may benefit most from the helping role. Although the stoma patient may have good health and few functional problems with the stoma or appliance, this is not necessarily congruent with acceptance of the stoma. In a study undertaken by Trainor (1981) she demonstrated that visitors had a greater acceptance of their stoma than the non visitor. Age, sex, type of stoma, length of time since surgery did not make any difference to the self-help visitor who had a stoma. The helping role encourages the visitor to expand social networks and helps with their confidence and self-esteem. It may be possible that the role of visitor in a self-help group is instrumental in helping some patients to come to terms with their stomas.

The Ileostomy and Internal Pouch support group

The Ileostomy Association was formed in 1956 by a group of patients and medical professionals as a mutual aid association with the primary aim of helping people who have had their colon removed. It was the first ostomy association in the UK and is a registered charity. At the first meeting, held at Birmingham General Hospital, 47 people were present and laid the foundation stone of the Ileostomy Association. The association adopted as its symbol the phoenix, a legendary Arabian bird worshipped in ancient Egypt, which burnt itself out every 500 years and rose rejuvenated from the ashes.

Since the recent advances in surgery such as the ileal–anal pouch, this group of patients has been taken into the Ileostomy Association, and the association has incorporated the words 'internal pouch' into its title.

The aims of the support group are to help people who have had an ileostomy or pouch surgery, and to help them adjust to their new body image and function. The confidence of many patients is dented after surgery and they feel that everyone knows about their new body image. Help and support is offered through the support group in the areas of rehabilitation, resumption of social activities, relationships with family and friends, employers, colleagues and the general public. The support group and its local groups aim to work in close cooperation with medical authorities as part of a team whose main aim is the rehabilitation of the ileostomy patient. Support is given to medical research into all aspects of inflammatory bowel disease and life with a stoma, with the aim of improving knowledge and reviewing and encouraging developments in new equipment and skin care products.

The activities of the support group are varied and meetings are arranged at regular intervals around the country by the group's divisions and branches. At these meetings there is usually a stoma care nurse or medical adviser with whom members can discuss problems. There will often be a guest speaker or discussion on a point of interest or medical subject. Ostomy manufacturers are invited to attend these meetings and there will usually be a small display with the representatives from the manufacturer who cover the area. A quarterly journal is sent to members which allows an exchange of views and advertisements of equipment with the facility to send for samples. Not all patients live in towns or urban communities and many are living in isolated areas in the UK. For them the journal proves a useful life-line and contact. Hospital and home visiting play an important part in the support group's activities. The aim is to give the new patient confidence and encouragement by showing them that someone has been through the same as they have and that life carries on. There are advisory services available on matters such as employment, housing, pensions, financial difficulties, insurance, marriage, pregnancy and sexual problems. There is support and counselling for the gay and bisexual man who is about to have, or has just had an ileostomy. For those members who travel abroad, central office can give details of a full cover policy that is available.

It is the policy of the association that all the officers of the national committee and local committees (apart from medical advisers) shall have ileostomies or internal pouches themselves and have a full understanding of all that is involved with an ileostomy or internal pouch. There are 60 groups locally throughout the country and one postal group. Full membership is available to anyone who has an ileostomy or internal pouch and patients should be given information when surgery is planned so that they can contact the support group if that is their wish. Associate membership is available to anyone who is interested in the association's work such as surgeons, doctors, nurses, social workers, friends and relatives.

The support group can be contacted at:
Tel: 01724-720150/0800-0184724
Fax: 01725-721601
E-mail: ia@ileostomypouch.demon.co.uk

The Urostomy Association

The Urostomy Association was established in 1971 at the Christie Hospital and Holt Radium Institute, Manchester, with 25 members and two company representatives. At that time there were very few urostomy appliances for patients and no stoma care nurses as they are known today. There was little interest from the medical staff, who were sceptical about whether the association would succeed. By 1972 the Manchester group had grown and a postal branch was established. In 1983 a new president took over, Clive Young, a urological surgeon with a positive commitment towards people with stomas. In 1984 the association changed its name from the Urinary Conduit Association (UCA) to the simpler Urostomy Association, the name by which it is known today.

The aims and objectives of the association are fairly wide-ranging, covering many aspects of a person's life. The association gives assistance in any way it can, both before operation and after, with counselling, help and advice regarding housing, work and marital problems, and helping patients to resume as full a life as possible.

The association is administered by a national executive, but each branch holds its own local meetings two or three times a year, to which guest speakers are invited to talk on medical and non medical subjects. Advice is also available from stoma care nurses. Appliance manufacturers attend and there is usually a small display of products with samples.

An association visitor will see patients in hospital pre- and postoperatively, on request, and appropriately trained visitors are able to undertake home visiting. There is a twice yearly UA journal distributed to all members and to postal members.

Full membership is open to all patients who have a urinary diversion such as a urostomy or continent diversion, and associate membership is open to those who have an interest in the association. Postal membership is not confined to the UK, and there are postal members in Ireland, Europe, Australia and South Africa.

The Urostomy Association can be contacted at:
Tel/Fax: 0245-224294

National Advisory Service for Parents of Children with a Stoma (NASPCS)

The NASPCS was formed by Sue Bird after her son was born with an imperforate anus. He was operated on a few hours after birth and given a colostomy which was a great shock to his mother. In the rural area where she lived the hospital had never dealt with a child with a colostomy before. Until the baby's reversal operation 6 months later, life was a nightmare. His mother had to cope with the fact that the baby had part of his intestines showing externally on his abdomen and there were no colostomy bags to put over the stoma. The hospital had said that

there were no stoma bags available for babies. It was a continual fight to stop the skin becoming sore and there was continual washing of clothes and bedding from the faecal output. When the baby returned for the reversal at Great Ormond Street Hospital, in the preoperative days a colostomy bag was used.

From this experience, Sue Bird decided that she would do all she could to prevent other parents going through the distress that she had endured. The foundations of a support group took shape and grew and literature was produced to help the parents of children with stomas.

The NASPCS is set up to provide parents of children with stomas with support and a contact point and to give information. It will give support and advice to parents of children with a variety of handicaps including imperforate anus, Hirschprung's disease and other disorders that lead to colostomy, ileostomy or urostomy.

They can be contacted at:
Tel: 01560-22024

The National Association for Colitis and Crohn's Disease (NACC)

The National Association for Colitis and Crohn's disease (NACC) offers support to patients who have been diagnosed with these illnesses and now has over 24 000 members nation-wide.

NACC has three main purposes:

- To give information through newsletters and booklets
- To offer support to both patients and their families through area groups. These groups hold meetings for members and their friends. Some meetings are social, at others specialists provide the latest news on medicines, diets and treatment. The association also offers support through a welfare fund for those in great need, and through NACC-in-Contact, which provides trained, supportive listeners available by telephone
- To raise money for research.

Membership of NACC is open to everyone with these illnesses, their relatives and friends, and health professionals.

The NACC service for members has the following free booklets, written by specialist medical advisers in non technical terms:

- Crohn's disease
- Ulcerative colitis
- The role of diet
- Medical terms used in IBD
- Drugs used in UC and CD
- Pregnancy in inflammatory bowel disease
- Inflammatory bowel disease in childhood
- Living with inflammatory bowel disease
- Can't wait card – this is a card that is accepted by numerous companies and large multiple stores, which, when shown, asks that the holder be allowed to use the toilet facilities urgently, as the holder has an illness which is not infectious.

Further contact can be made via:
Tel: 01727-844296

The British Colostomy Association (BCA)

Under the auspices of the King's Fund for London in 1963, a pilot scheme was organised at the Royal Marsden Hospital with funding from the King's Fund, to ascertain whether there was a need for some form of group or association relating to patients who had cancer and surgery resulting in a colostomy. After the initial pilot survey in London, a decision was taken to establish a charity for the benefit of providing guidance and assistance to colostomy patients in the UK to help with rehabilitation and to enable them to have a better quality of life. The association became a registered charity in September 1966.

After achieving registration, the Colostomy Welfare Group (CWG), as the new charity was then called, became a national organisation providing guidance, advice, care and assistance in rehabilitation to colostomy patients throughout the UK.

The financing of the Colostomy Welfare Group in 1972 was taken over by the trustees of the Cancer Relief Macmillan Fund, and it was decided that the CWG would provide services to colostomy patients in the UK, and Cancer Relief would provide the necessary funding to achieve that objective without the CWG being a separate charity appealing for funds. This enabled CWG to increase initiatives across the country to enable area organisers and voluntary visitors to give a service to colostomy patients.

In the 1980s the CWG became the British Colostomy Association (BCA) with headquarters in Reading and 25 individual areas across the UK, providing a service to at least 20 000 members each year. Since 1994 the BCA has striven to ensure that colostomy patients anywhere in the UK have access and help at 24 hours notice, 7 days a week.

The volunteers who work with BCA all have a colostomy and therefore have the necessary skills and experience to inspire and help new patients. Volunteers do not counsel but have training and ability to give practical support and encouragement and non medical information.

Patients can contact the BCA and area organisers contact a volunteer in the area to assist with the patient request. Volunteers are often recruited because of the help they received when recovering from stoma surgery or are recommended by stoma care nurses.

The association does not organise regular self-help group meetings as the ileostomy group does, but area organisers can arrange open day meetings where patients can attend and ostomy manufacturers will be present with their products. Often stoma care nurses arrange patient open days and the local BCA area is invited to meet new patients.

Any patient who contacts the BCA will be assured of complete confidentiality and for many patients in rural areas it proves invaluable. A telephone and letter help line is part of the BCA service, along with a wide range of literature to help and support the patient. Basic information on colostomy is also available in:

- Spanish
- Greek
- Polish
- Punjabi
- Gujurati.

The BCA is at:
Tel: 01734-391537

Hidden problems in stoma care

18

Paediatric stoma care

STOMAS IN INFANTS AND CHILDREN

A stoma in a neonate, whether as an emergency procedure or as an elective procedure, can be extremely distressing for the parents, especially if it is needed because of congenital malformation. The stoma in the neonate is often temporary, whereas the stoma in the older child may be permanent. Approximately 300 stomas per year are raised in children under the age of 1 year. Overall, 80% of paediatric stomas are raised in babies in the first 6 weeks of life, 10% up to the first year of life and 10% in children over the age of 1 year (Webster 1985). The majority of the stomas are colostomies, but some children will require ileostomy and a few a urostomy. Because the skin of preterm infants is more permeable, there is likely to be increased absorption via the skin. There is also a greater ratio of surface area to body weight and chemicals in skin care products can be absorbed through the skin. The epidermis can be easily traumatised and the stratum corneum is only partially effective as a barrier and can be easily damaged. As the infant's gestational age increases, the preterm infant's skin becomes similar to an adults.

When an infant has a stoma raised there are special considerations that should be taken into account when the nurse is caring for the infant. One-piece appliances are most suitable and are light-weight. It must be remembered that a young baby will find a two-piece appliance heavy and cumbersome, and even with a light-weight paediatric appliance on a very tiny preterm infant (usually less than 2 kg) the appliance can be heavy enough to cause difficulty with the infant's breathing, taking into account all the other tubes and devices that are attached to preterm infants in an incubator. Often the easiest way of caring for a faecal stoma in a very small preterm infant is to use petroleum jelly around the peristomal area skin and lightly cover the stoma in gauze with a layer of petroleum jelly on the gauze and to frequently change the dressing. Once the infant's condition becomes more stable, a light-weight paediatric bag may be used. During the care of the infant in the special care baby unit the parents are taught about the care of the stoma and how to change the appliance. Parents often worry that taking the appliance off hurts the infant and re-assurance must be given to parents that it is quite safe to change the appliance once or twice a day and it will not harm the infant. Liaison with the community paediatric team and the infant's health visitor enable all the caring agencies involved to understand each other's role and also their limitations. The stoma care nurse in a district general hospital will probably see very few paediatric stomas each year and will not be a paediatric trained nurse, so will have limited experience of general paediatric care, therefore liaison with the other team members enables the team to care for the infant in a holistic manner.

Most parents and nurses become very worried when they see the stoma discolour to either bluish or white when the infant is crying. This happens because infants usually pulls up their knees and contract the abdominal muscles when crying and the bowel is momentarily trapped by the contracted muscle. Once the infant stops crying the stoma returns to its usual colour. Changing the appliance is often easier if two people are present, especially if the infant is crying. While one person changes the appliance the other can try and distract the infant. Parents should have a good routine for changing the appliance and make sure everything that is needed for a pouch change is ready beforehand, with the appliance cut to the correct aperture size. As the infant grows and starts to toddle a two-piece appliance may be more appropriate and easier for the parent to manage. Being inquisitive, the toddler may want to pull the appliance off at various times. If the toddler still needs nappies this will help to hold the appliance in place, and clothes such as dungarees help stop the toddler from removing the appliance at inappropriate times and places.

As the child with a stoma reaches school age there may need to be a discussion with the school and nursery carers or school welfare worker about the care of the stoma and any help the child may require. A closed appliance may be easier for a nursery child to manage than an appliance with a clip. A one-piece appliance may make it easier for the child to be self-caring with a little supervision from the welfare worker. Privacy for the child should be established in the matter of toilet and washing facilities. A normal parental attitude to the child with a stoma helps the child to develop a normal body image

CONGENITAL DISORDERS

For the neonate who requires a stoma after birth, the majority are temporary stomas and are done because there are congenital disorders which manifest themselves in the first few days of life and may be life-threatening. The most common of these are Hirschprung's disease, imperforate anus and malrotation of the gut.

Hirschprung's disease

Hirschprung's disease occurs in approximately 1 in 5000 births and causes intestinal obstruction. There is an absence of ganglion cells in the distal colon causing lack of innervation of that particular part of the bowel section. In approximately 80% of neonates with Hirschprung's disease the problem is located in the rectum and sigmoid areas. As the part of the gut lacks innervation, intestinal obstruction occurs between the normal and abnormal segments of bowel. It may not be picked up until a few days after birth and if the disease is present in a mild form, diagnosis can be delayed until the child is older. For some, diagnosis is not established until later in life. In approximately 25% of neonates with Hirschprung's disease it is diagnosed with intestinal obstruction, abdominal distension and vomiting.

The treatment plan is to relieve the intestinal obstruction and at a suitable later date to restore bowel continuity. The obstruction is bypassed and a loop transverse colostomy is raised. The colostomy is left in situ until the infant starts to thrive and definitive surgery is done about the age of 6 months to 1 year. After this toilet training can begin in the normal way.

Anorectal malformations

One of the common anorectal malformations seen is that of imperforate anus. Anorectal malformations occur in about 1 in 5000 births and are slightly more common in males. These malformations often occur with other defects that can be classified as low, intermediate or high defects. Low defects lie below the pelvic musculature and can often be repaired by a local perineal operative procedure. High lesions occur above the pelvic floor musculature and require extensive surgery. Intermediate lesions come between both of these (Hampton & Bryant 1992).

Imperforate anus is identified immediately after birth as the midwife tries to take the infant's temperature rectally and is unable to do so. Immediate surgical intervention is needed to create a diversion, usually through a loop colostomy, and then further radiological investigations or fistulograms will be needed to define the extent of the lesion. After surgical correction of the low or high lesion the stoma is reversed and a new anal opening is created. The parent is taught how to do anal dilations at home to maintain patency of the anal opening, and these dilations have to continue for several months. Over the years many of these children experience constipation or diarrhoea and parents should be reassured and given help and advice, especially during the toilet training years. Some babies born with imperforate anus can now benefit from advances in surgery which allow posterior sagittal anorectoplasty as early as 3 months, with closure of the colostomy a few weeks later. It is thought that these children have an improved chance of continence when toilet training starts (Johnson 1992).

Malrotations

Malrotation is an abnormality in the rotation of the midgut and its mesentery which happens during foetal development and which may result in severe complications. With malrotation there are often other congenital malformations, including prune belly, anorectal malformations, Hirschprung's disease and biliary and oesophageal atresia.

Treatment consists of assessment of the ischaemia of the bowel and resection of the necrotic bowel with the possibility of a stoma. There may also be volvulus and intussusception which require surgery.

Necrotising enterocolitis

Necrotising enterocolitis (NEC) is predominantly seen in the preterm neonate and has a mortality of 30–50%. NEC is an acute necrosis of the gut involving the area of the distal terminal ileum. On rare occasions the whole of the ileum and colon may be affected. NEC occurs because the bowel has become injured through an ischaemic event such as birth asphyxia, congenital heart disease or damage of the bowel mucosa by feeding formulas. Perforation of the bowel wall may occur.

Gastrointestinal symptoms of NEC include abdominal distension, retention of formula, ileus and bloody diarrhoea. If NEC is suspected, feeding is stopped and a nasogastric tube is passed to decompress the bowel. Any accompanying infections are dealt with appropriately. If the acute attack resolves the feeding is slowly restored and the infant carefully watched for further recurrence. If there is an indication that the bowel is gangrenous or has perforated, surgical intervention will be necessary. Laparotomy and resection of the bowel and a proximal stoma is the procedure of choice. Of the infants who survive medical and surgical management of NEC, 10% will need surgical intervention at a later date to relieve the intestinal strictures that develop.

Intestinal obstruction

Obstruction of the bowel may be due to dynamic or adynamic reasons. Obstructions that are adynamic are often due to the absence of bowel peristalsis resulting in paralytic ileus. Factors that contribute to adynamic obstruction are previous abdominal surgery, medication, spinal disease, metabolic dysfunction or injury. Many resolve on their own accord or when the initiating cause is removed.

Dynamic obstruction of the bowel can be due to a pathological condition and may become a surgical emergency. Dynamic obstruction in the bowel can be due to Crohn's disease, adhesions from previous surgery, a strangulated hernia or malignancy.

Obstruction is usually sudden in onset with little warning. There may be vomiting and lack of stool or flatus. Abdominal X-ray will show dilated loops of small bowel and distended large bowel with an absence of gas distal to the obstruction. Perforation is the serious complication of obstruction and a nasogastric tube is passed to relieve nausea and pain. Surgical intervention diagnoses and corrects the underlying cause and a stoma proximal to the cause may be needed.

Meconium ileus

Meconium ileus accounts for 15% of neonatal small bowel obstruction and can be seen associated with other paediatric intestinal problems such as Hirschprung's disease. Infants with fibrocystic disease of the pancreas are likely to exhibit the symptoms of meconium ileus and it is the most serious of the gastrointestinal symptoms of cystic fibrosis (Johnson 1992). The meconium in the proximal ileum may induce intestinal obstruction, perforation or gangrene of the bowel. Often the problem can be corrected by using preparations to wet the meconium or by emulsifying the meconium with a preparation such as a hyperosmolar enema (Gastrografin®). Surgical intervention is needed if dilution of the meconium plug is unsuccessful. The bowel is dissected and reanastomosed. A temporary ileostomy may be needed. The ileostomy would be a double-barrelled stoma allowing access distally to the meconium plug and the ability to use further hyperosmolar enemas to help dissipate the plug and clear the distal bowel.

Faecal incontinence

For various reasons, some children are incontinent of faeces and as the child becomes older and starts school this can become difficult and embarrassing. For these children there is a form of management to help them have some control over the bowel. This is colonic irrigation. Based on the same principles as irrigation of a colostomy, it can be taught to the child and be done while sitting on the toilet. When the procedure is finished the child can be clean for up to 48 hours.

The ACE procedure (antegrade colonic enema) is a new surgical alternative for children who soil or experience severe constipation. The appendix is used and tunnelled out through the abdominal wall as a small opening which is catheterised and an enema solution is distilled followed by normal saline. This produces evacuation of the colon and can last up to 48 hours (Johnson 1992).

Paediatric nursing in itself is a specialised area and babies with a stoma are often cared for by a paediatric trained stoma care nurse. Within the UK, only three paediatric centres offer a stoma care nursing service. Many of the babies with very specialised needs will be cared for in a children's hospital such as Great Ormond Street Hospital in London and the Alder Hey Children's Hospital in the north of England. Here there are stoma care nurses fully aware of the needs of this group of patients.

Further in depth reading on pathophysiology and diagnostic studies of gastrointestinal tract disorders and paediatrics can be found in *Ostomies and Continent Diversions: Nursing Management* (Hampton & Bryant 1992).

19

The elderly ostomate

Problems with stoma care are increased dramatically for the older ostomate. Care becomes more difficult as there are often more physical demands and incapacities to cope with and these may be accompanied by loss of one or more faculties. Today the average life expectancy is 83 years for men and 87 years for women. Certain areas of the UK, especially on the south coast of England, have high populations of people over the age of 70 years (the national average in most areas of the UK of people over 65 years is 15.3%, but in some of these south coast areas the average is as high as 27.9%). By the year 2000, 10.6% of the population of the UK will be over the age of 80 years. For many of these patients there are already other long-standing physical problems which are going to be further complicated by stoma surgery. These problems include:

- Parkinson's disease
- Alzheimer's disease
- Huntington's chorea
- Cerebral vascular accidents
- Chronic obstructive airways disease
- Blindness or impaired vision
- Deafness
- Mental ill health
- Loss of upper or lower limbs (one or both)
- Multiple sclerosis
- Heart disease
- Arthritis.

With the incidence of cancer of the colon and rectum and diverticular disease, and their complications, being greater in the elderly, patients in their 80s and 90s undergoing major surgery often see it as the final threat to their independence and as something which will make their lives more difficult. In recent years there has been more publicity in the media about colorectal surgery and stomas, and both elderly patients and their relatives are more aware of the reasons for this type of surgery and the benefits in terms of improving health or possible prolongation of life. Although the aims and goals for recovery after stoma surgery are the same for the elderly patient, there are particular challenges in communication skills and ingenuity for the stoma therapist.

Among some of the early problems the nurse, doctor and stoma therapist will encounter are the increased fear of dependence which may, perhaps, lead the patient to reject surgery. The family too may be reluctant, as they may fear that the ageing relative may have to come to live with them, or that they are going to be asked by hospital staff to take some role in the care of the relative. Family support and acceptance of the ostomate are essential for the successful rehabilitation of the patient and the discharge back into the community to their home or wherever they wish to go and live. At a time of crisis like this patients may say that they will sell their home and move into sheltered accommodation or into a nursing home, as they will not be able to manage any more. At this stage patients must be discouraged from making wide sweeping, life changing decisions until they have had a chance to go back home and assess the situation. If patients feel that they will not be able to manage their stoma care, a family member may be willing to help and work with the nurses and stoma therapist to enable the stroke handicapped, arthritic or visually handicapped patient to remain independent. It must never be presumed that spouses will automatically help and care for patients without first fully discussing all the implications with them.

For some patients the admission for gut surgery may be the first time that they have been in hospital undergoing major surgery and it can be an intimidating and upsetting time for them. It can be difficult for them to comprehend and adjust to the changes in their routine and environment, and for some patients who are admitted as an emergency, they may well be debilitated and confused because they have been ill for a few days at home prior to routine or emergency admission. In hospital they may well find themselves in a bed with cot sides and next to a stranger. They do not understand why they cannot get out of bed alone and have to ring a bell for assistance. Often with poor hearing and postoperative confusion there is difficulty in understanding medical staff and explanations. Many have great difficulty in understanding ward staff who are from ethnic minorities and some patients can be rude to these staff because of cultural difficulties. Faced with the loss of basic bodily functions and disrupted routines, elderly patients may feel as though they have regressed to childhood and become tearful or aggressive.

For patients to recover, it is best if they can take control in the situation and if procedures are as uncomplicated as possible. Although the ability to learn does not always diminish with age, patients need time to assimilate new skills and adjust to the change in their excretory habits. Time, patience and repetition are needed by ward staff to teach the elderly patient self-care and sometimes it can be frustrating for both staff member and patient. Often what has been taught the day before is forgotten the next day. A chair and a full length mirror are useful to enable patients to sit down and to see their full abdomen in the mirror to learn self-care. A mirror often helps patients to make the breakthrough in self-acceptance of their changed body image as well as enabling them to be independent with self-care. It is advisable to remind patients to check their appliances from time to time to ensure there are no leaks. Older patients often have a reduced sense of smell and would be mortally embarrassed if they felt that staff, family, friends and neighbours thought that they smelled.

Physical appearance is still important to older patients, although they are less likely than younger ostomates to worry about the appliance showing through tight, short clothing. They are often more comfortable in looser fitting clothes under which an appliance is less noticeable. Some women like to wear a girdle and it will be

loving relationship that is given to the ostomist. The spouse or partner can often act as the main supportive crutch through the pre- and post-operative period into the rehabilitation period, helping the patient to make a good psychological and physiological recovery. Probably the biggest problem the ostomist has to face is the emotional one and the emotional response that comes from the partner and the spouse, but surveys have shown that patients do need help and advice with sexual and psychosexual problems after stoma surgery.

Stoma care nurses are in a unique position to establish a close rapport with their patients which enables them to explore the patients' inner fears and thoughts. The nurse is able fully to explain the effects of the stoma surgery in relation to the patient's sexual relationship and self-esteem.

Patients having a stoma for malignant disease have been found to be more concerned about the disease process than about the stoma and stoma care nurses should be aware of the priorities set by patients and their families at the time of crisis. The four major concerns have been found to be:

- Fear of the cancer spreading
- Needing to have further treatment
- Fear of death
- Having cancer.

In research it was found that 70% of participants ranked concerns differently from their spouses, showing the need to assess both partners separately (Krumm 1982). Both patients and spouses rated concerns to do with sexuality lower than expected therefore anticipating the question that professionals are focusing on perceived issues rather than on patients' actual concerns. Concerns relating to sexuality become more of a priority later in the recovery period when the patient has rehabilitated in the community and life is beginning to return to normality.

CONTRACEPTION AND PREGNANCY

Discussion should take place with ileostomy patients of child-bearing age regarding the future choice of contraception and pregnancy. Mechanical methods such as the cap, condom and intrauterine coil are safe to use. Female patients who want to use the coil as a method of contraception and who have had extensive bowel surgery that may have involved the vaginal wall (with possible scar tissue involvement), may need to discuss this with the gynaecologist and surgeon.

The female patient with an ileostomy who wants to use oral contraceptives should be made aware of absorption via the gut, especially if a large amount of small bowel has been removed. Some of these young women will have had amenorrhoea during their inflammatory bowel disease period and it may be a while before their periods return. These patients should discuss with their doctor the advisability of starting the pill before their periods return. Low dose oral contraceptives are often not adequately absorbed in women who have had a colectomy with ileostomy and their margin of safety is reduced (Todd 1978).

Pregnancy is not contraindicated after stoma surgery, but advice is often given to wait at least a year to allow scar tissue to heal and if the patient has had inflammatory bowel disease for many years prior to surgery, a wait of 2 years may be advised. Problems that may occur include displacement of the stoma by the enlarging uterus and abdomen, causing difficulty in seeing and changing the appliance. In nearly all cases vaginal delivery is possible, but women who have undergone panproctocolectomy may need a careful episiotomy due to perineal scarring. For these women, discussion between surgeon and obstetrician can be beneficial. Changes in hormone balance can alter the adhesiveness of the appliance, and some women find that the appliance does not adhere as well as it used to when they were not pregnant. Conversely, some women may find that the appliance is more sticky than normal. As the abdomen starts to swell to accommodate the growing baby a change to a different type of appliance may help. Patients who wear a two-piece appliance may find that this becomes too rigid and one of the softer one-piece appliances is easier to manage. With the growing abdomen the stoma may retract into the abdomen and changing to an appliance that is convex may help to push the stoma out and stop leakage under the flange. A belt with a convex appliance may be useful. Convex appliances should only be used under the guidance of the stoma therapist. If not used circumspectly, they may cause damage to the stoma. Patients have reported that after giving birth the stoma returns to normal, with some mothers stating that the stoma has improved, especially if it was a stoma that retracted causing undermining of the appliance. Women with colostomies who go through a pregnancy often report constipation and their dietary intake should be examined. Both colostomates and ileostomates need to take adequate fluid during pregnancy, and sleeping on the side away from the stoma often helps relieve the pressure on the stoma. A few pregnancies sit uncomfortably on the old surgical site and stretch the old adhesions. This can cause cramps and pain and these can be misdiagnosed as early labour if the woman is admitted to hospital and medical staff are unaware of her previous surgical history. For women who have ileal–anal pouch surgery and do not have an ileostomy, the obstetrician should be fully aware of the patient's reformed anatomy internally, especially if there is any likelihood of a Caesarian section being performed. Discussion with the surgeon who performed the pouch surgery would be useful so that the obstetrician can understand the new internal arrangement of the small bowel (Black 1988, 1994c).

GENDER DIVERSITY

A neglected issue in stoma surgery and stoma care is the patient who is homosexual. Gender diversity is more evident in contemporary society, but there is still the idea of heterosexual dominance in society, medicine and the health care systems of the country (Taylor & Robertson 1994, Eliason 1993). As previously seen, nurses often find difficulty in discussing patients' sexual needs and homosexual and bisexual patients facing stoma surgery, whether temporary or permanent, are doubly disadvantaged.

The preoperative counselling of this group of patients is important if they are to make a full emotional recovery after surgery and return to their communities to lead a normal and productive life. Therefore the therapeutic relationship between the nurse and patient is made on the first contact. There are medical terms for gay male sexual activities, but it will be unlikely that the patient will be aware of these and the forming of the therapeutic relationship is founded on the language that the nurse uses and that the patient is familiar with and understands. It is important that the person counselling the gay male before and after stoma surgery negotiates the most appropriate form of language. Some nurses and doctors who hold negative attitudes to homosexual patients will find that they are hampered by their lack of awareness and sympathy with these patients' needs. It is possible for the nurse or doctor to make the appropriate attitudinal shift, but this cannot happen before there is acknowledgement of prejudices that are held.

In the course of counselling, sexual activities are likely to come up and the nurse should be aware of the appropriate terms that will be used. Once trust has been set up the homosexual patient may wish to discuss more particular experiences and fantasies. A major impact for homosexual men is surgery that requires removal of the rectum, such as an abdoperineal resection resulting in a colostomy, or panproctocolectomy resulting in an ileostomy. Health care professionals often presume and use the stereotype of gay sex as being one active partner and one passive partner, which is often not the case. It is common for both men in a relationship to switch roles in penetrative anal intercourse. After this type of surgery one of the problems will be that while the man will probably be able to continue with penetrative intercourse the reverse will not be so. If this is not fully explained in preoperative counselling to both partners, an emotional imbalance in the relationship occurs with the possible breakdown of the relationship. There is recorded evidence of suicide after stoma surgery, abuse of the newly repaired perineal area, abuse of the stoma, social isolation, psychological breakdown and self-mutilation of the stoma (Devlin et al 1971; Black 1988, 1994c).

The needs of bisexual patients are often ignored in the health care environment, especially those patients undergoing stoma surgery. This group of patients may have a heterosexual partnership that is long term, but also have other casual partnerships of either sex. The sexual identity of these patients may cause difficulties because of their lifestyle, and this type of relationship may be very difficult for nurses to cope with while at the same time having a good therapeutic relationship with the patient. For this small group of patients undergoing stoma surgery, it may be necessary to involve another health professional who is at ease with the patient's type of lifestyle.

Helping gay men to understand and mourn the death of part of their sexuality empowers them to move on. They may find that there are pressures to renounce their sexual needs entirely but this should be resisted. Stoma surgery is invariably life saving so should not spell the end of sexuality. It may well be that if a homosexual man perceives that he will encounter homophobic treatment in his health care, he will request a second opinion in order to find a surgeon who would provide more professional treatment. In today's health service nurses and doctors have to acknowledge the existence of a patient's sexuality, whatever it may be, so that holistic care may be given.

21

Multicultural issues in stoma care

In today's multicultural society there are implications for the nurses and doctors who provide the health care services for that society. During training, nurses have been taught to consider the individual and his or her needs, the individual's family, and the social context in which the appropriate health care is provided. The cornerstone of this caring has been the Western biomedical model which focuses on symptoms and their assessment, history, treatment regime, evaluation and follow through. Awareness and understanding of the multicultural world in which the nurse works and ways of knowing people in different frames of reference is challenging and nurses are beginning to recognise the values and beliefs and health practices of different cultures in order to provide culturally appropriate care that is relevant to this population.

Capra (1982) suggests that being aware of this new cultural movement requires new research and the evolution of new conceptual models.

The new vision of reality we have been talking about is based on awareness of the essential interrelatedness and interdependendence of all phenomena—physical, psychological, social and cultural. It transcends current disciplinary and conceptual boundaries and will be pursued within new institutions. At present there is no well established framework, either conceptual or institutional, that would accommodate the formulation of the new paradigm, but the outlines of such framework are already being shaped by many individuals, communities, and networks that are developing new ways of thinking and organising themselves according to new principles.

Nurses are beginning to realise that apart from the obvious fact that many patients from ethnic minorities have little or no command of the English language, religion and customs affect the ways in which patients perceive their care. The environmental context in which individuals have been reared may influence health perceptions and health influences. Culture and ethnicity may influence one's physical development and exposure to health compromising environments and conditions. Culture may also influence the family structure and how individuals respond to health and illness.

For nurses to provide culturally competent care – a complex integration of skills, knowledge and attitudes that cross cultural communication – they must demonstrate respect for others and promote the well-being of the patient. Although a comparatively small number of stoma patients come from ethnic minority groups, a failure by nursing and medical staff to understand their special needs can lead to isolation of individuals on returning to their community, indeed in some circumstances they may become outcasts of that society. Smaje (1995) suggests that the contemporary ethnic character of Britain's population was forged in the 19th and 20th centuries, largely as a result of government policies. Black and minority ethnic people have made their home in Britain for many decades, and the patterns of migration have evolved the demographic structure of communities that is seen in Britain today. The 1991 census figures show that 3 million people in Britain are from black and ethnic communities. The largest proportion of the 'black' community is from India, with the next largest from the Caribbean followed by Pakistan. At its inception in 1948, the founding principle of the National Health Service was the provision of appropriate and accessible health care to the population of Britain. The wide ethnic diversity now seen brings to the forefront the need for the NHS to respond appropriately, with cultural and clinical competence, in the provision of care for these groups which until now have occupied a marginal position when it has come to health policy and delivery.

In delivering appropriate and culturally competent care health care, providers and educators must increase the understanding of beliefs and practices and values that are relevant to different cultural groups. Not only should the needs of the ethnic minority patient be considered but also the needs of ethnic minority learners. Bonarparte (1979) suggested that often nursing is taught and practised as if all patients were members of the dominant Christian, Caucasian group, and as a result the potential therapeutic interaction between nurse and patient is often handicapped by a tendency for the nurse to have ethnocentric beliefs about the superiority of Western health standards.

The main barriers and anxieties of ethnic minority patients in seeking the health care and services they require are:

• Colour
• Communication
• Culture
• Customs
• Religion.

Skin colour is often perceived to be the biggest barrier to be overcome and insensitivity by health care workers reinforces this perception. Gloves may be put on before examination takes place and in stoma care conducted by ward staff gloves are used when cleaning the stoma and replacing the appliance, so conveying to patients that they may have an infection. If no contact is made by the health care staff, it may be inferred that there is racial discrimination.

Communication can be a major hurdle in helping people from ethnic minorities. Some speak very little English or no English at all. Patients from Pakistan will speak Urdu or Punjabi. Patients from Bangladesh speak Bengali, patients from Gujarat will speak Gujurati, Hindi or Kutchi, and East African Asians will speak Swahili or English. Patients from the Caribbean will speak English but may follow their own patois.

Asian patients will often come from two different continents. Some will come as first generation migrants from the Asian continent and some will have migrated to the African continent and then have come to Britain after the Ugandan conflict. South Asian patients will have kept their own cultural health beliefs and traditions, whereas those from the African continent will have been more influenced by Western culture. Patients from the Afro-Caribbean countries hold their own traditional beliefs and ethos. Many will be from the second or third generations to be born in Britain and so will be well acquainted with the health care system and aware of how to access the services they need. But even for these patients there is the worry that local health care will not understand some of their cultural needs. These patients are often more at ease and have a better rapport with health care providers from an Asian background than with Caucasian health care providers.

Most Asian patients from Pakistan, Bangladesh and East Africa are of the Muslim faith. Patients from Gujarat will be predominantly Hindu or Jain, those from Arab countries are almost invariably Muslims, and some East African Asians follow the Buddhist, Sikh or Christian faiths. For each of these faiths there is a culture and customs which often affect the way patients perceive their health care and the way in which they dress and what they eat. These ways often do not fit neatly into the routine of the NHS and this is where conflict can occur if health care professionals are not aware of the cultural needs of their patients.

The Hindu patient

Hinduism has many gods and goddesses, who are the manifestations of one God. Hinduism is a very diverse religion and is considered more a way of life than a religion. There is no standard form of worship and some Hindus pray, some meditate, some practise yoga and many combine all of these. Although there are Hindu temples, many people worship at home at a small shrine in which there is a statue or image. Some Hindus like to fast once a week and this should be discussed with Hindu patients, particularly those with an ileostomy. There are no particular attitudes to clothing, although Hindu women may wear a sari. They are also modest and may be reluctant to undress or allow a male nurse or doctor to examine them. Some strict Hindu men will not allow their wives to be seen by male health care professionals at all. In general surgery this may cause difficulties, as most consultant general surgeons are men and indeed the whole surgical team may be male. For surgical procedures, Hindu women should be offered two X-ray or operating gowns to wear, one in the normal manner and one to go over the top with the opening at the front so that their back is not exposed. Long hair is very important to Hindu women and they may not cut their hair without their husband's permission.

Hindu patients will not eat anything that comes from or is made from cattle as they believe that the cow is sacred. Some are vegans and will not take medication that has a gelatine capsule or eat jelly. This can cause problems in Hindu patients who need to take Imodium® to slow bowel transit time down as the medication comes in capsule form. With awareness, health care staff can substitute the medication in syrup form, so avoid causing conflict for the patient. Other forms of food that can help in thickening bowel output are marshmallows and Jelly Babies, but these also contain gelatine. Less orthodox Hindus may be prepared to take Imodium capsules as it is seen as medication to help them recover. Such matters should be fully explored on admission of the patient so that problems are not encountered.

Consent to treatment of any kind using the statutory legal requirements is sufficient, but female patients may need to consult their husbands or the husband may want to be there when the consent is signed.

Jainism is an ascetic Indian religion older than Buddhism which is very strict and austere, and few Jains are found outside India. They are strict vegans and do not harm living creatures. Help in understanding these patients' needs can be obtained from the local Hindu temple.

The Sikh patient

Sikhism developed in India in the 16th century. It includes much of the teachings that are common to Hindus and Muslims. The Sikh's belief is based on teachings from ten gurus, the last of whom died at the beginning of the 18th century. A Sikh must be baptised according to Sikh rites and must be able to read and write Punjabi. He must always defend his religion and carry a weapon, the *kirpan* (now symbolic), and this requirement may cause difficulty when the patient wishes to keep it with him in hospital and even go to the operating theatre with it.

Sikhs have five religious symbols, known as the five Ks. These are:

- Uncut hair – *kes*
- The comb – *kangha*
- The steel bangle – *kara*
- The dagger – *kirpan*
- White shorts – *kacha*.

Sikhs should not have their hair cut or bodily hair removed unless it is really necessary and then only a minimum should be removed. The small comb is kept in the hair under the turban and Sikhs must wear a steel bangle on their wrist. Often there can be problems in carrying the ceremonial dagger and a symbolic one may be worn. The white shorts are worn as underwear by the men and they like to continue wearing them in hospital if at all possible. Sikh women wear a sari or long dress and will often wear a head scarf. Many Sikh women will prefer to be examined by a female health care professional if at all possible. Many Sikhs prefer not to eat beef and may refuse medication unless it is really necessary.

The Muslim patient

Islam is the religion followed by Muslims and its holy book is the Koran. A Muslim is expected to pray at set hours, five times per day, and before each prayer session has to perform *al-wadhu* (a washing ritual). The washing signifies cleanliness of the body inside and out, and this ritual can be difficult for the patient with a stoma.

In 1987, the Fatwa Commission was petitioned for a ruling on Muslim stoma patients in regard to ritual prayer. The commission was told that at the time of prayer the patient is unable to change the appliance, and asked whether it was possible for patients to pray while carrying excrement. In answer to this question it was stated that as

the stomal output cannot be controlled, stoma patients may perform *al-wadhu* at the onset of the prayer interval and may pray as many times as they wish during this interval.

At the onset of a new prayer interval the ablution performed previously is not valid and the patient must perform new ablutions. In such cases a two-piece stoma appliance is essential as it allows a clean pouch to be attached to the flange at each new prayer interval, thereby leaving the patient clean and pure for prayer (Black 1994c).

At preoperative counselling the culture and religion of the patient should be ascertained correctly, so that discussion can take place about his or her future needs regarding their religion after surgery. If the patient undertakes *sujud* (prostration for prayer) a secure appliance is vital. It must also be remembered that Muslim patients are very particular about cleanliness, and faeces are considered unclean. Siting the stoma below the umbilicus in Muslim patients would cause extreme distress, with the possibility that the patient would not be willing to undertake self-care. A stoma sited above the umbilicus is viewed as food content that is being put out and therefore acceptable for the patient to self-care. (For the Caucasian patient a stoma situated above the umbilicus is difficult to manage as the natural waist line is near the umbilical area.) Another factor to consider with Muslim patients is that the right hand is used for eating and greeting and the left hand is used for cleansing oneself. A majority of the population is right-handed, and it is often very difficult for them to carry out intimate care with the left hand. Once again careful preoperative counselling will elucidate whether the patient follows this ritual. If so, careful thought is necessary to determine which appliance will be the easier to use. The obvious type is a one-piece appliance with a pre-cut hole that can be managed single-handed. A flange with a pouch that has to be clipped on is difficult to manage with one hand (which in addition may not be the dominant hand), and problems such as leakage and falling off may occur.

To Sh'ite Muslims from desert regions, having the stoma cleansed by the nurse using tissues or wipes is anathema. This group of patients are used to cleaning themselves with sand or stone in the desert and they opt not to use tissues or wipes. This may cause a problem when a flange needs cleaning and the easiest solution is to shower off faeces from the flange or skin. If this is a problem, using a large syringe filled with water and squirting around the flange or stoma will enable the patient to clean the area (Black 1988, 1994b).

Some of the areas that can cause cultural conflict with Asian patients and health care professionals are listed in Box 21.1.

Muslim patients, like Hindus and Sikhs, may be vegan or vegetarian and not eat beef in any form. For them, on first seeing a stoma, especially an ileostomy, it may appear to be like a piece of raw steak, and they will be aghast. In the early days of convalescence vegetarian patients with a stoma will find that the vegetable rice that is often the mainstay of their diet causes flatus and pain. Removal of legumes and peppers will often only leave white rice and chapati and such a diet will increase stomal output, causing dehydration and bringing about lack of protein for tissue repair. Well meaning advice for dietary prohibitions can lead to a cultural conflict for the patient and his or her carer.

Box 21.1 Potential areas of conflict or misunderstanding with Asian patients

Food and diet
- Acceptable or forbidden foods
- Preparation and hygiene, serving and eating

Personal hygiene
- Methods of cleansing
- Preparation for meals and prayers
- Male: shaving
- Female: menstruation, pregnancy and preoperative depilation

Social
- Mixed sex wards
- Operation consent
- Medical/nursing examination by opposite sex

Body image
- Response to disfigurement

Death, dying, bereavement and grief
- Religious laws, attitudes to death, needs of relatives, preparation of body for disposal

---

The Muslim or Hindu patient may enquire about the make-up of the flange or the adhesive on the appliance, and whether they contain animal products that may not be acceptable to them. Knowledge of the constituents of the adhesives will ensure that the Muslim or Hindu patient is not offended or upset.

Religious requirements

Religion plays an important part in the life and culture of ethnic minorities, and for the Muslim stoma patient there can be significant problems, particularly during Ramadan. Ramadan occurs in the 9th month of the Muslim calendar and each year Muslims observe a period of fasting from dawn to dusk. During fasting they are not allowed to drink even water and exemption is only allowed during illness and long distance travel.

The ileostomy patient is particularly affected by Ramadan as a 12-hour period without fluid can cause dehydration, especially in manual workers in the warmer months. Again, good and knowledgeable preoperative counselling of how religious feasts and fasts may affect the stoma patient is of vital importance. Because it would be dangerous to go without fluid for a long period, it is not unknown for the patient to go and discuss this with his Imam (learned religious man). In complicated situations such as this may be, the GP, stoma care nurse and surgeon should give medical advice and the patient should discuss religious clarification with the Imam.

Problems may also occur because the patient overeats at *sehri*, the meal taken before sunrise in anticipation of the next day's fasting. Pseudo obstruction of the stoma may occur if incorrect foods have been consumed. Problems that may be experienced by Muslim colostomy patients during Ramadan include constipation and perhaps nausea caused by lack of fluid, leading to the drying out of the stool in the colon. Overeating at *sehri* may cause continual diarrhoea in the following 24 hours. In the urostomy patient it is vital that the consequences of fluid withdrawal are fully understood, including the fact that renal problems may occur if fluid is severely restricted.

The month in which Ramadan falls varies from year to year and when it occurs during the summer months the sunrise to sunset period can be extremely long. Eating is only allowed after sunset, which can be as late as 10 p.m. Because of the extended family many Asian patients may live in substandard housing stock that is shared with Western families. Here problems can arise with the preparation of *sehri* as often kitchen facilities are shared and this can disturb other tenants when cooking takes place late in the evening. In such situations the patient may resort to convenience food or junk food or even go without their only meal of the day.

Further disruption of the stomal output may occur due to over-reaction of the ileostomy or colostomy output. Disruption of day time work and night time rest will result from the patient having to empty or change the appliance more frequently (Black 1992).

Some health care workers from ethnic minority groups may have religious and cultural cognitive dissonance in caring for stoma patients. In some cases the revulsion may be so deep that it violates their belief to help in the care of the stoma patient. This should be considered by the ward manager and, if necessary, the health care worker allocated to care for other patients. Spector (1977) suggested that it is not sufficient to direct the nurse to be non-judgemental and accept the person for what he or she is. The nurse will require guidance to reach full appreciation of the patient's needs in respect of his or her own culture if the nurse is to provide truly individualised care.

Translation for non English-speaking Asians may be a problem. As noted earlier in this chapter, there are several languages commonly spoken in the subcontinent, with many dialects. It is entirely inappropriate to ask the hospital domestic worker to translate for the patient because they speak the same language. The Asian patient is an extremely private person and does not welcome discussion of his or her welfare by someone outside the family. Elimination is not something any of us would want to discuss with

someone we do not know, therefore efforts must be made to find a medical translator who is acceptable to the patient and his or her family. Most hospitals and hospital switchboards keep a list of approved translators from within the hospital and also from approved translating services. Occasionally if the translator is from a non approved source, the translation of what the patient needs to know does not take place. The translator may feel that what the patient is being told is not what the patient needs to hear, leading to problems when unexpected surgery takes place. Repercussions from this lack of understanding can be extreme, especially if the patient does not realise that a stoma is the eventual outcome of the proposed surgery.

It would be impossible for health care workers to expect fully to understand all the cultural and religious needs of the ethnic community that they come into contact with, but they should at least be aware of the make-up of their local community and have some idea of what possible problems may occur when these patients are admitted to hospital. Key points to remember in caring for patients from ethnic communities are:

- Know which country the patient comes from and which religion they follow
- Understand how major feasts and fasts would affect the patient
- Appreciate the patient's need for prayer at set times, which may be disruptive to ward routine
- Understand dietary considerations
- Be aware of translation needs
- Have a structured management plan
- Make sure there is a cultural awareness among other health care providers in the team
- Ensure that the service is culturally, psychosocially sensitive.

Limited translated leaflets for Punjabi and Gujurati speaking patients who are about to have a stoma are available from the Ileostomy Association and the British Colostomy Association.

22

Travel and holidays

Many people who have stoma operations feel in the early days after surgery that they will never be able to travel far from home or be able to go on holiday again. A few patients make a plan that as soon as they are well enough they will go away on holiday to enjoy their new beginning. Going on holiday and travelling should not present a problem for those with a stoma, and should be just the same as without a stoma. By taking a little more time to think about what the individual with a stoma will need and remembering a few important points, he or she should be able to enjoy a happy holiday.

Many patients, particularly those who had inflammatory bowel disease before stoma surgery, will be a little apprehensive about travelling to foreign countries – they will remember what it was like travelling when they had inflammatory bowel disease and the difficulty there could be in finding toilet facilities, especially toilets that were reasonably clean. These memories and the thought that they may have to change their appliance fills them with horror, so, they reason, the best way to avoid these problems is not to travel. However, provided advice is sought and taken and a few useful reminders adhered to, there is no reason that the stoma patient should not travel, either within the UK or abroad, with the minimum amount of trouble.

Before travelling

In the early days after surgery it is sensible to start with small trips away from home to build up confidence and to be sure that the appliance is secure and safe. A few weeks before travelling, contact with the local stoma care nurse will enable the patient to discuss any problems that may arise while travelling. The stoma care nurse will also be able to give patients travelling abroad a travel certificate in several European languages that inform customs that the patient has a medical condition that may cause embarrassment if the appliance is disturbed. If the stoma works on a regular basis the patient will know when to change the appliance, but an ileostomy will need regular emptying as will a urostomy. Travelling by car enables the route to be planned to allow for comfort stops at regular intervals where there are adequate toilet facilities. Motorway and shopping centres have disabled toilets which are kept locked and a key for these can be obtained at minimal cost to enable the patient to use facilities that give more space and also washing facilities that are private. (Keys are available from RADAR – see Appendix.) If travelling by rail, sea, air or coach there are usually adequate toilet facilities, although they may be a little cramped.

Travel insurance is important if travelling abroad, but it is important to ensure that the policy does not exclude pre-existing conditions (i.e. a medical condition that existed before the date of effecting the policy). Patients are able to check on travel insurance queries from their local appropriate stoma voluntary organisation. The Ileostomy Association can give details of full cover travel policies for patients with ileostomies. Also it is important that the patient checks whether the country to be visited has reciprocal arrangements with the NHS.

On the journey

When travelling patients should keep all their ostomy supplies with them at all times, and when flying supplies must never be put in the luggage hold, but must always go as hand luggage. Some airlines allow extra hand luggage for medical supplies and this is always worth checking with the airline when making a booking. When going abroad patients should take double

the amount they would normally need to allow for bowel upsets due to change in water and food and long haul travel and the possibility of being delayed unexpectedly.

Patients should be told how to make up and travel with a small holdall that will contain the supplies essential for changing en route if the need arises. In this kit it is useful to have a small bottle of water or cleansing wipes to use while on the move.

If travelling by air, luggage may be searched and inspected and the use of the travel certificate helps customs to understand that embarrassment can be caused if the patient's bags are searched in public. By booking an aisle seat, patients who have an abdominal perineal resection are able to stretch their legs and change their position if seat belts have to be kept on. Also a seat near the toilets enables the patient to use the facilities before food is served and the queues for the toilets start. The change in air pressure on an aircraft affects everyone, whether they have a stoma or not, and this can be minimised by avoiding carbonated drinks and eating regularly. It may be preferable to wear a two-piece appliance while travelling as this can be 'burped', but today there are ileostomy bags with filters that act in the same way as filters on a colostomy bag. Some patients use inflammable solvents to clean peristomal skin or to remove the stoma appliance. These cannot be carried on an aircraft, but the local chemist or stoma care nurse should be able to advise a suitable alternative. When travelling by sea or air a stoma appliance change may be necessary. Many of the ostomy companies now do a specially adapted travel bag that has several pockets, a hook, mirror and scissors. These can be obtained from the stoma care nurse or the ostomy company.

Patients who travel by car must wear a seat belt. A properly fitted and adjusted seat belt will not cause harm or damage to the stoma. Any involvement in an accident will cause less damage, both to the stoma and the patient, if a seat belt is worn. If the seat belt feels uncomfortable and lies across the stoma, a commercial device that fits to inertia seat belts is available from any good car accessory shop. It allows the seat belt to be worn loosely while driving, but on undue braking the seat belt recoils and locks in the normal manner. Patients still unwilling to wear a seat belt may ask their GP for an exemption. If the GP endorses it, the patient will be charged a fee. The motor insurance company must be informed of the endorsement and the insurance cost may rise to take account of the endorsement.

Food and drink

In the UK and abroad nearly all hotel and boarding house accommodation now has en suite facilities, making appliance changing on holiday less embarrassing. Patients travelling to hot countries should be advised that appliances should be kept as cool as possible so that the adhesive does not melt. Keeping the appliances in a cool shady position is adequate – they should not be kept in a refrigerator.

As with any holiday abroad, whether the patient has a stoma or not, care should be taken with food and water consumption. Ice cubes and salads should be avoided as local water is often used. Food that appears to have been left out in the heat for a long time should be avoided. Exotic food should be taken in moderation and foods that disagreed with the patient at home will continue to do so. If travelling long haul the patient should be advised to acclimatise slowly in the first few days, spend only moderate amounts of time in the sunshine and keep up the fluid levels. Bottled water should be used, with the seal intact. Fruit should be eaten in moderation as excessive amounts may cause diarrhoea. It is useful for colostomists and ileostomists to take antidiarrhoeal preparations away with them and understand how to take them.

Patients who irrigate should take the same precautions with the water they use as they do with the water they drink. Still bottled water is advisable for irrigating. Alcohol can be drunk, but over indulgence causes problems with being unable to care for the appliance properly and can also cause dehydration.

On the beach

Patients who have a stoma and go away for a beach holiday feel that they will be unable to swim, either in the sea or pool, because of their stoma. They can, however, swim in a pool or in the sea, but must at all times wear a pouch over the stoma.

Swimwear may pose a difficulty and a stoma high on the waistline in men may cause difficulty in finding suitable swimming apparel. High waisted trunks such as boxer shorts are ideal and ordinary swimming trunks can be worn underneath. For women, swimming costumes with a sash or bow on the same side as the stoma help to disguise any bulges. Costumes with big patterns help to distract the eye. Swimwear is available from small companies specialising in clothes for stoma patients, but often something suitable can be found in high street stores. Colostomy patients may be able to wear a leisure pouch over their stoma for sports activities.

Networking

Across the world, in nearly every country, a stoma care nurse or company or agent contact can usually be found. The first worry of stoma patients venturing abroad is what will happen if they lose their appliances or need practical help. A few weeks before leaving, the stoma care nurse should be contacted. The nurse will be able to give the patient a stoma care nurse contact or, if there is not a nurse available, one of the major ostomy companies will be able to give an agent or company number. These companies have free telephone helplines (see Appendix for a list of numbers).

23

Healthy eating

Many of the worries of patients are about food. Both patients and their relatives are frequently under the misapprehension that only certain foods are allowed and that they will have to be on a strict diet. Ostomists soon discover, once they start eating again, that there is a relationship between their food and fluid intake and their stomal output. The elderly patient who is on a restricted income worries about the cost of the correct type of food. Many young patients prefer a fast food diet without enough natural fibre. So what is the best way of eating for the new ostomist, and for the many patients for whom this will be a way of life for many years to come? In proffering dietary advice to patients, nurses must consider patients' economic situation and give advice that patients will be able to follow sensibly and economically, also taking into account any medical conditions, such as diabetes, that will preclude the intake of certain foods.

Regular excretion and consistency of excreta contribute to easy management of the stoma. Since a disciplined intake of food enables the patient to have more control over gut function, there is an advantage in suggesting to the patient that a few guidelines should be followed:

- Avoid undereating
- Eat little and often after the early days of surgery
- Achieve a nutritionally balanced diet
- Have a food intake that is high in natural fibre
- Food that causes excessive flatus should be taken in moderation

- After the rehabilitation period, eat three meals a day at regular times.

Body weight is important as fluctuations can affect the stoma and the diameter of the stoma, therefore affecting the appliance aperture, so the patient should be encouraged to try and maintain a fairly constant weight. If the patient is overweight, weight loss should be achieved by a slow and steady loss and not by crash dieting. Loss should be no more than 1 kg per week so that the peristomal skin is able to adjust. In patients who are underweight, fast weight gain may cause the stoma to retract.

Ileostomies

For many ileostomists, the adjustment to being able to eat normally after recovery from surgery is quite difficult. Many patients have given up dairy products before surgery in an attempt to control their disease and are not used to eating high fibre foods or fruit with pips (Farbrother 1993). The output from an ileostomy will never be as firm as the output from a colostomy – on a good day the output may be of a 'porridgy' consistency and on a bad day the output will be very fluid, necessitating many trips to the bathroom to empty the appliance. What constitutes a bad day or a good day? The body's biorhythms can be upset by many things which are not connected to dietary intake. Anxiety over something such as a hospital appointment, an argument, a general feeling of being ill (not necessarily physiological) or just generally feeling down.

Apart from a balanced dietary intake, ileostomists needs to drink at least 2.5–3 litres per day of fluid (De Ridder 1997). Ileostomists pass about 400–800 g of effluent per day and about 600 ml of this is water. The important constituent in this output is salt (around 4 g per day) that is lost by the body. Other nutrients such as potassium, calcium, magnesium, iron, zinc, fat and protein are equal to that lost by the large bowel. The majority of ileostomists have enough salt occurring naturally in their diet (8–10 mg) and any unwanted salt is excreted in the urine. Most of the salt taken in the average diet is added to processed food by the manufacturers, while 10% is naturally occurring and we add 15% during cooking or at the table. If an ileostomist's output is more than 1000 g per day there is the danger that salt and water may be inadequate. Many patients exhibit subclinical salt depletion in the form of listlessness, irritability, tiredness, weight loss and diarrhoea. When diarrhoea occurs there may be vomiting and excessive perspiring as in the case of fever, or if the weather is very hot and exercise has been taken, the salt and water reserves need to be brought back up to the normal level as quickly as possible with salted food such as crisps, soups or salted vegetables. A simple rehydration drink of salt and sugar – ¼ teaspoon of salt and 1 teaspoon of sugar in a glass of water – can help. Other useful and palatable home prepared drinks that have a salt content are Oxo and tomato juice and fruit juices for potassium replacement. Proprietary rehydration products such as Dioralyte® and Rehidrat® are useful as a standby. The main causes of acute ileostomy diarrhoea are:

- Food poisoning
- Abdominal infections and abscess
- Viral infections
- Obstruction.

Kidney stones are more common in people with ileostomies than in the general population. Stones occur because the urine of a patient with an ileostomy is more acid than normal and there is smaller volume which makes circumstances suitable for the precipitation of calcium urate in the kidneys. People with ileostomies who live in hot climates and undertake a lot of sport may need extra salt in their diet.

Among the factors which control the amount of ileostomy output are the amount of small bowel left after surgery and the health of the small intestine, especially in the presence of Crohn's disease. The short-term factors controlling ileostomy output are diarrhoea, food containing excessive dietary fibre, stress and salt taken on its own.

Foods that help to thicken ileostomy output are:

- Porridge (using proper oats)
- Shredded Wheat

- White rice and white rice water
- Smooth peanut butter
- Stewed apple
- Marshmallows
- Jelly Babies
- Root vegetables, especially potatoes
- Bananas when they are underripe, before the starch is converted into sugars
- Brown bread
- Cream crackers.

Patients with an ileal–anal pouch may find that anal irritation is one of their biggest problems. This is caused by the frequent passage of effluent which will be very like the output that ileostomists produce. Eating late in the evening and eating large meals irregularly increases the need to evacuate the pouch, with the associated continual disturbance of the sleep pattern. Continuing the eating pattern that was started when the patient had an ileostomy will help the pouch patient with the ileal–anal output. Although with an ileostomy certain fibrous foods such as celery, nuts and unpeeled apples may cause a blockage of the stoma, these may be adequately expelled in the patient with an ileal–anal pouch. Nuts or very nutty cereals may cause a problem to the pouch patient as they may scratch the pouch as they pass through, causing severe pain for which nothing can be administered. Time will heal the scratched area in the pouch and analgesia may give relief.

Laxatives are not needed for a patient with an ileostomy, but patients who like mint sweets may have a problem with diarrhoea as often these are sweetened with a sugar substitute called sorbitol which acts as a laxative. Some foods and cakes are also sweetened with sorbitol. Anyone with an ileostomy needs to be careful in the early postoperative days but should be able to return to a full normal and balanced diet, only avoiding foods and drinks that they know cause problems.

Colostomies

There are fewer dietary problems for the patient with a left-sided colostomy as, with time, after the postoperative period, the stomal output should become formed. Patients should be advised to eat little and often rather than one or two big meals per day. It must be remembered that many colostomy patients are in the older age groups and find a change in their eating patterns hard to understand. For older patients, to be asked to 'graze' through the day rather than have three big meals is difficult, as many have been brought up to only eat at regular times and not to eat between meals. Many also will have changed to white bread after the Second World War and find it strange to be asked to eat brown bread. Most colostomy patients need little help or guidance on what to eat to help their stomal output, and when questioned many are found to have a well-balanced diet within their economic means.

The patient with a colostomy will need a nutritional intake that is high in natural fibre and this includes foods such as:

- Porridge oats
- Shredded Wheat
- Root vegetables
- Underripe bananas
- White rice
- Brown bread.

Sometimes the colostomy patient may suffer from constipation. This often happens in the elderly patient, who may fluctuate from constipation to diarrhoea. Laxatives such as lactulose are often prescribed, but eating a kiwi fruit on a daily basis will often help to relieve constipation. Elderly patients are often on other medications which may have a constipating effect and this must be borne in mind when the nurse is investigating the cause of the constipation. Older patients will sometimes suffer from urinary incontinence, either as a result of their surgery or through the gradual passage of time. Patients who are liable to be incontinent sometimes restrict their fluid intake considerably and this may be a cause of constipation. They should be encouraged to increase their fluid intake and ways of helping with the incontinence investigated. Patients questioned about their fluid intake will often assure the nurse that they are drinking enough. When questioned more closely they are found to be drinking large amounts of tea and coffee. Tea and coffee contain caffeine which is a diuretic and causes the patient to lose more fluid, and, in addition, caffeine predisposes towards constipation. The diuresis causes thirst and this is quenched with more tea and coffee, so perpetuating the cycle. It is far better for the patient to drink more water, if necessary with diluted squash in it.

Patients who have had diverticulitis for many years and have restricted their diet to soft foods to help prevent colicky pain sometimes find it very difficult to re-educate their eating patterns after having a colostomy and eat more high fibre foods. They also feel that they should continue to avoid fruit with pips in, which further restricts their nutritional intake. If saliva is hard to stimulate, causing difficulty in mastication and the feeling of not wanting to eat as everything tastes of cotton wool, a slice of lemon sucked 20 minutes before a meal helps with the stimulation of saliva and gastric juices. The main problem in encouraging effective eating is re-educating the patient, and some simple advice is often all that is needed:

• Take your time to eat and do not let yourself be rushed
• Prepare everything that you need before you sit down to eat
• Eat slowly and chew everything well
• Try to drink before and after meals and not with the meal (drinking with eating causes air to be gulped, so causing wind and discomfort).

Urostomies

Patients who have a urostomy raised should be able to follow a normal pattern of eating once they have recovered from the surgery. The main concern for this group of patients is an adequate intake of fluid. Potassium should be encouraged in the form of potatoes and bananas and there may be the need for extra potassium to be prescribed by the doctor. The urine may become alkaline which leads to problems of skin irritation and urinary tract infections. The pH of the urine should be kept between 5 and 7. Taking 100 mg ascorbic acid daily helps to absorb much of the

mucus that the conduit produces, so making the urine look clearer. Another side-effect of ascorbic acid is that the excess that the body does not need is excreted via the urinary system making the urine appear to be a golden colour. Also recommended is cranberry juice which acts as a bacteriostatic and helps with the intake of vitamin C. Again the economic situation of the patient must be taken into consideration as cranberry juice is quite expensive and a litre a week is needed. GPs will sometimes give ascorbic acid on prescription.

It is necessary for patients with a urostomy to have a high fluid intake (2.5–3 litres of fluid per day). Many of these patients have had radiotherapy before their surgery and this will often have an effect on bowel function. Many find that after urostomy they experience a long period of diarrhoea and help with understanding what the correct foods are will aid their recovery. Likewise here, marshmallows and Jelly Babies help to thicken output. Dietary manipulation, as in the ileostomy patient, will be effective. Particular foods that cause problems with urostomy patients are asparagus, which makes the urine smell (see also Box 23.1), and beetroot, which colours the urine red causing the patient to believe that there is blood in the urine. If urostomy patients are constipated after surgery, purging laxatives such as senna should not be given as there is a risk of the bowel sutures coming loose. If a laxative is needed, something gentle such as lactulose is suitable, and kiwi fruit daily. Kiwi is also very high in vitamin C which helps with tissue repair.

Methane and hydrogen sulphide gases produced by the bowel during the digestive process build up and are usually known as gas, wind, flatus or flatulence (see also Box 23.1). Whatever we decide to call it, all human beings have flatus and it is responsible for faecal odours. Some patients with ileostomies have a lot of flatus while others have little. It is the same for colostomists. For the patient with a stoma and appliance, the bag may blow up like a balloon and cause social embarrassment. Today there are colostomy and ileostomy appliances with good filtration systems and it is a case of finding the one that is best for a particular patient and his or her circumstances.

Yoghurt and buttermilk are useful components of meals since they help to reduce flatus and odours. They are particularly helpful when the patient has to take antibiotics and help to replace some of the bowel flora (Black 1988). Foods that can contribute to the problem of flatus are baked beans, onions, chewing gum, pulses, sprouts and drinks such as carbonated drinks, beers and lagers (see also Box 23.1).

Dieting

Some people with stomas feel that they need to lose weight at some time in their lives, just as people without stomas do, but ostomists often think that they should not diet as it may harm their stoma. This is not true, but before starting on any weight loss diet patients should consult their doctor and talk with their stoma care nurse. Unless there are specific reasons, any of the dieting books or clubs are suitable. The important point to remember is that crash diets are unsuitable. They are popular because weight loss can be fast, but very quickly the weight is put back on. Crash diets may also upset patients' metabolism, causing problems with stomal output. In addition, skipping meals and reducing the intake of fluid can cause dehydration and an imbalance of electrolytes. The method that doctors and dieticians recommend is the slow and steady way, aiming to lose 1 kg per week. Weight lost this way is likely to stay off, but it does mean that calories have to limited. With this type of weight loss the patient can plan meals ahead and if there is a food that the patient and his or her stoma cannot tolerate this can be avoided. Even diets like these need willpower and it often helps to join a club with like minded people.

Box 23.1   Foods causing problems following surgery

The following foods may cause problems for stoma patients after surgery. It must be remembered, however, that the foods listed may also cause problems for people who do not have a stoma. It is only in the early weeks after surgery that patients should be wary of foods causing wind as they may also cause pain as the wind passes through the anastomosed bowel.

Foods that may cause flatulence
Pulses, nuts, citrus fruit, mushrooms, chewing gum, onions, sprouts, peppers, leeks, garlic, shallots, cucumber. Carbonated drinks, beers and lagers

Foods that may cause odour
Asparagus, eggs, fish, onions, pulses, vitamin B tablets, leeks, melon, mushrooms, garlic

Constipating food
Maize, muesli, popcorn, almonds, asparagus, mushrooms, pulses, sugar

Foods causing anal irritation
Raspberries, strawberries, fatty foods, spices, groundnuts, citrus fruit, alcohol

24

Pharmacological considerations

For some stoma patients, prescribed and over the counter drugs may have unwanted and unpleasant side-effects on the gut and may alter the stomal output. Increase in the ileostomy output may lead to dehydration, and alteration in colostomy function may lead to constipation. It is therefore important for nurses, community nurses and stoma care nurses to understand what effect their patients' medication may have on the stoma.

Drugs affecting stomal function can be divided into three groups:

1. Drugs that can affect the function of the gut via the autonomic nervous system (one of the most powerful systems to affect gut action), such as:
   — cholinergic drugs
   — adrenergic drugs.
2. Drugs that have a direct action independent of the autonomic nervous system, such as:
   — analgesics
   — antibiotics
   — laxatives
   — antacids
   — ion-exchange resin.
3. Drugs that have an indirect action on the gut, such as:
   — sedatives
   — diuretics
   — digoxin.

When the parasympathetic system is stimulated it produces increased peristaltic activity causing a rise in secretions and a relaxation of the sphincters that may cause diarrhoea. Drugs such as noradrenaline and dopamine – used with some patients with a stoma in the intensive therapy unit – will have some effect on their gut action. Noradrenaline decreases peristalsis and may cause constriction of the gut sphincters and dopamine may cause a decrease in peristaltic action.

Anticholinergic drugs exert their effects on the gut via the cholinergic receptor sysytem and atropine is a classic example. Atropine is found in Lomotil® which is used to control gut motility. Examples of anticholinergic drugs are:

- Atropine
- Belladonna
- Dicyclomine
- Hyoscine
- Propantheline.

There are also a number of drugs that may be thought not to have an effect on the gut but which are likely to cause gut disturbance. The main ones are the tricyclic antidepressants, which include:

- Amitriptyline
- Desipramine
- Dothiepin
- Doxepin
- Maprotiline
- Nortriptyline
- Protriptyline
- Trimipramine.

All the above drugs have an anticholinergic effect on the gut. Some antidysrhythmic drugs used for abnormal heart rhythm have profound anticholinergic effects, producing dryness of the mouth, slow micturition and constipation. Most sedating antihistaminic drugs have anticholinergic side-effects and may cause constipation. Commonly these drugs are used for people who suffer from hay fever. The following are some of the frequently used antihistamines:

- Brompheniramine
- Chlorpheniramine
- Cyclizine
- Cyproheptadine
- Diphenhydramine
- Dimenhydrinate
- Promethazine.

Monoamine oxidase inhibitors have similar effects to sympathomimetics and can cause constipation.

Laxatives come in many varieties and their main effect is to increase stool frequency. Osmotic laxatives increase the fluid volume of the stool. Bulk laxatives increase the consistency of the stool. Lubricant laxatives do as their name suggests, they facilitate the passage of the stool through the bowel, and stimulant laxatives are thought to act on the neuronal plexus in the wall of the gut (see also Box 24.1).

Constipating drugs include antacids containing divalent and trivalent, some of the narcotic drugs such as morphine and its derivatives codeine, dihydrocodeine and diphenoxylate. Distalgesic® is a popular analgesic in gut surgery and although it contains dextropropoxyphene it is less constipating than the previous analgesics.

Antacids containing magnesium cause diarrhoea, especially if taken in large quantities. Antibiotics are well known to cause diarrhoea, especially tetracycline and ampicillin which disturb the micro-organisms in the gut. Drugs taken for hyperlipidaemia will cause diarrhoea as the action is to remove bile salts which are responsible for fat emulsification.

Box 24.1   Laxatives

Solid bulk laxatives
Agar
Bran
Frangula
Ispaghula
Methylcellulose
Psyllium
Sterculia

Osmotic laxatives
Lactulose
Magnesium salts
Sodium salts

Lubricant laxatives
Dioctyl sodium sulphosuccinate
Liquid paraffin

Stimulant laxatives
Senna, cascara, danthron
Bisacodyl
Phenolphthalein

Whole tablets are sometimes seen in the patient's stoma appliance when emptying it, especially in ileostomy appliances as there is not the facility to make formed stools. This will often worry patients who think they are not receiving their medication and the nurse should reassure the patient. Some drugs are formulated with a wax matrix and the impregnated drug in the matrix is leached out during the passage of the drug through the gut. The most common modified release tablets are:

- Burinex K®
- Centyl K®

- Esidrex K®
- Navidrex K®.

If the stoma patient's drug regime has recently been changed there is a strong possibility that it may be one of the drugs that is responsible for the disruption of the gut, even though it is believed that the particular drug under normal circumstances would not disrupt gut action. It should always be remembered that almost any drug can upset the gut in one way or another

Ethics and research in stoma care

25

Role and development of the stoma care nurse

HISTORY

As described in Chapter 5, in reviewing the literature we find that the history of bowel disease and associated surgical procedures can be traced back to Biblical times. Pre-Christian Israelites were aware of the consequences of the spillage of 'dirt' after abdominal injuries (see also Ch. 5). The earliest recorded milestone in stoma surgery was made by Heister, who described the perfection of enterostomy operations on battle casualties in Flanders in 1707. William Cheselden was said to have been one of the first surgeons to help form a colostomy in 1756. Later, in the time of the Napoleonic wars, Dominic Larrey expounded that injured bowel should be exteriorised to allow the faeces to pass out of the abdomen. Present-day procedures began to be developed in the 19th and early 20th centuries (Black 1994a).

In 1944, an ileostomy was performed by Strauss on a young chemistry student called Koenig. At that time there were no suitable appliances for stomas and Strauss had told the patient there would be the need to catch the effluent from the stoma on a continual basis. Koenig was interested in mechanics as well as chemistry and developed a bag suitable for himself that fixed to the skin with a latex preparation, and in 1947 the Koenig Rutzen stoma bag was introduced to the UK (Strauss & Strauss 1944). In 1950, Brooke devised the everted ileostomy which prevented stricture and helped in the development of better ileostomy appliances.

From the middle of the 19th century to the present day, the basic concept of colostomy construction has remained unchanged. Hartmann in 1923 described elective resection of rectosigmoid cancers with a left iliac fossa end colostomy, and Patey (1951) and Butler (1952) introduced the abdominoperineal resection for cancer with colocutaneous suturing and an extraperitoneal colostomy. The use of colocutaneous suturing and extraperitoneal colostomy helped overcome the problems resulting from stenosis or prolapse of the bowel which had caused many problems in earlier surgery (Black 1994a).

Until 30 years ago there appeared to be no suitable alternative to urinary diversion for malignancy and abnormalities of the bladder. Improvements on the early ileal conduits did not come until 1950 when Bricker devised and perfected his ileal conduit, which today is taken as the gold standard (Black 1994a). There are few historical milestones in the formation of continent pouches although Leaver (1993) states that urinary diversions were known as far back as the 19th century.

The first mention of stoma care is when Plumley (1939) described how a patient worked out his own care of his ileostomy as there was no one to tell him what to do. There were no professionals then and patients had to cope as best they could, relying on their own ideas about caring for themselves and talking with others who had been through the same experience. In reviewing the early literature on stoma surgery from the UK and USA in the 1940s and 1950s, it is clear that there were many social, psychological and physical problems associated with having a stoma (Lahey 1951, Patey 1951, Butler 1952, Strauss & Strauss 1944, Brooke 1952).

In the USA, in 1958, Norma Gill, who had undergone surgery for ulcerative colitis and had an ileostomy at the age of 34, vowed that if she survived her illness she would help other people in the same situation. Although neither a nurse nor medically trained, she was recruited by Dr Turnbull at the Cleveland Clinic as a stoma therapist and opened the door to a new nursing speciality. In 1961, with Dr Turnbull, the first training programme for professionals was set up

to teach them how to help stoma patients to adjust to their new way of life. Gill was instrumental in the organisation of the United Ostomy Association and the formation of the World Council of Enterostomal Therapists.

At about the same time, in 1966, in the West Midlands and Essex in the UK, stoma clinics were being run by former patients who helped and advised new patients. In 1969, at St Bartholomew's Hospital in London, a ward sister, Barbara Saunders, had seen the needs of patients who were having stoma surgery and the support that they required from a professional source, and set up a clinic with her surgeon Ian Todd. Referrals came in increasing numbers from surgeons, GPs and physicians and following discussions with the hospital, doctors and the DHSS, Barbara Saunders became the first stoma care nurse in the UK in 1971. Further discussion between the DHSS and the Joint Board of Clinical Nursing Studies (JBCNS) led to the first course in stoma care at St Bartholomew's Hospital in 1972, and trained nurses from the hospital and the community who wanted to work in the area of stoma care applied for the courses. The JBCNS (later the English National Board for Nursing, Midwifery and Health Visiting (ENB)) was among the first for identifying clinical specialities and developing post basic education.

In 1977 the Royal College of Nursing (RCN) formed the Stoma Care Forum to which nurses with an interest in stoma care or working in stoma care could belong. In 1978 the DHSS brought out a paper entitled *The Provision of Stoma Care* (Department of Health and Social Services 1978) which was intended for health authorities who were considering their stoma care arrangements and wanted to know about appointing a trained stoma care nurse to care for this group of patients. The paper emphasises the importance of good arrangements for providing information to patients with a stoma, and to the GPs about appliance requirements when the patient is discharged from hospital. The paper felt that patients with a stoma, although they form a small part of the health needs of a district, face a considerable problem in coming to terms with living with a stoma. The main needs for stoma care were seen as:

- Psychological preparation of patient and relatives before surgery where this is possible
- A suitably sited stoma, and the provision of an acceptable and well-fitting appliance
- Advice on the management of the stoma, the appliance and skin care
- Advice and psychological support over problems that may arise during recovery from surgery
- Continued care and advice after discharge from hospital in relation to any changes that may occur to the stoma and appliance.

Good practice and the organisation of stoma care suggested that in the development of a comprehensive service there should be a trained stoma care nurse in each health care district, based at the district general hospital, and the function of the stoma care nurse would be to ensure as far as possible continuity of care for the stoma patient in both hospital and the community. The stoma care nurse would hold a clinic to which patients could be referred for advice or appliance refitting. The clinic would run alongside the surgical clinic so that advice could be sought if necessary. The stoma care nurse would have close links with the GP and also be a resource for information for the primary health care team and local pharmacists. There would be an element of the job that would teach and advise hospital nurses, community nurses and other staff in the care of stoma patients. There would also be an element of research required in the role of stoma care.

The paper states that experience with stoma nursing posts has shown much improved service to patients. Additional costs can be offset by the savings achieved by the use of the correct appliance and expert evaluation of new equipment. The paper also suggested that it would be some time before a comprehensive service could be made available in all or even a majority of health districts.

In 1985, Lee suggested that although stoma care nursing had been identified only 15 years previously as a speciality, stoma care nurses were well thought of as a group within the nursing profession. In official documents of the RCN they are used as an example of a well-established element of the health care team, as practitioners who are of help to the patient. As a result of this rapid assimilation into the health care system there was the possibility that stoma care nurses could become complacent and a victim of their own success as a specialist group.

It was seen by far-sighted visionaries in 1985 that in the climate of change in the health service at that time, and the attitudes and opinions about the type of care that the health service should supply, stoma care nurses must be prepared to meet the challenges thrown up by the changes taking place. They would have to consider their role and possible budgeting restraints that changes in the health service would bring. Few if any stoma care nurses in 1985 had any idea where the change would be coming from and how it would affect them.

THE SPECIALIST NURSE

Over the last 20 years there has been considerable expansion of the role of the specialist nurse in the UK. Some of the earliest specialists, described in many articles, are stoma care nurse specialists. The role of the stoma care nurse specialist can be justified as meeting the needs of patients since generalist nurses have inadequate knowledge to deal with the specialised problems of stoma patients and the equipment they need. Wilson-Barnett (1995) suggests that these roles are often supported by the medical profession to relieve doctors' increasingly heavy burden, and the wider, more holistic approach to care is suitable for the nursing philosophy. Later specialist nursing posts are often created or supported through charitable (Macmillan) or soft (research or company) moneys, and once established are seen as essential to the patient group they serve. The RCN document *Specialities in Nursing* (1988) stated: 'Specialist practice involves a clinical and consultative role, teaching, management, research and the application of relevant nursing research. Only if a nurse is involved in all of these is he or she a specialist.'

Cost–benefit analyses in several studies of specialist nurses in different areas of nursing are able to demonstrate value in the care that they provide (Wilson-Barnett & Beech 1994, Montreux Study 1998, Zimmer et al 1984, 1985, McWinney 1994, Maule 1994, Hamric & Spross 1983). Consistently, it has been shown that where there are advanced levels of nursing skills they become associated with beneficial outcomes. Wade (1989), in a paper delivered to the International Nursing Congress in Seoul, found that a cost–benefit analysis of having a stoma care nurse could anticipate savings in the reduction of stay of hospitalised patients, continuity of care for patients and reductions in the amount of wasted equipment at hospital and community level.

The United Kingdom Central Council (UKCC 1994) has stated that a specialist practitioner demonstrates higher levels of clinical decision making and will be able to monitor and improve standards of care through supervision of practice, clinical audit, the provision of professional leadership and the development of practice through research, teaching and the support of professional colleagues. In an article by McSharry (1995) about the evolving role of the clinical nurse specialist, it is suggested that the rise in clinical nurse specialists is because there is a perceived need to manage resources effectively, to initiate research, and to promote interaction with education in the clinical setting.

Various writers have suggested what the role of the clinical nurse specialist should be for particular patient groups (Gowers 1981, Castledine 1982, Miller 1995). Castledine, between 1981 and 1983, conducted research into the role of the specialist nurse and identified eleven characteristics, although Gowers (1981) had defined the characteristics as being in only four main areas. Miller (1995) described five main areas. However, all three writers had a common theme. The role of the specialist nurse is divided here into five areas:

• Clinical expert
• Researcher
• Consultant
• Teacher
• Change agent.

These paint a broad picture of the role the clinical nurse specialist undertakes. The precise role will depend on management expectations, patient and staff expectations and the nurse's own professional development and aims. In examining the impact that the clinical nurse specialist makes on a particular patient or client group, two areas need to be analysed:

1. How the clinical nurse specialist affects patient outcomes
2. How the specialist role interacts with general nursing practice (Markham 1988).

By 1985, it was being suggested by Williams & Johnston (1983), MacDonald et al (1984), Devlin (1985) and others that stoma care nurses had not fulfilled the earlier higher expectations that the DOH (1978) paper had suggested they might. Even with the research by Wade & Moyer (1989) there appears to be very little published research examining patient outcomes. Wade (1989), in *A Stoma is for Life*, found that patients in stoma care nurse districts were likely to be more satisfied with their appliances and not experience as many problems as patients in non stoma care nurse districts. Patients with stoma care nurse involvement were happier with their knowledge about their condition, satisfied with the care they received and able to look after themselves and their appliances. But in 1995, Notter was still worryingly suggesting that the role of the clinical nurse specialist needs further research to show the measurable effect that is made on patient outcomes.

SPONSORSHIP IN STOMA CARE

In 1985, when Lee suggested that stoma care nurses should rise and meet the challenges of the changing provisions of health care, little did she realise from which direction one of stoma care's biggest challenges would come. In 1989 there were rumblings among stoma care nurses and the ostomy industry about sponsorship of stoma care posts. This was something quite new to the health service and no one was sure what this was about or how it would work.

By 1990, the Stoma Care Forum at the RCN felt that the subject should be put to congress in the form of a resolution to be voted on as to the way forward. The resolution asked that council examine the current position of health care agencies entering into sponsorship arrangements with private companies and take the appropriate action to persuade such agencies to abandon these arrangements where the independent judgement of the nurse is compromised. The resolution stated that there was considerable anxiety among nurses and patients, who believed that the NHS was being commercialised at the expense of putting the patient first. If nurses have their judgement compromised by interested party sponsorship, are they still able to provide a comprehensive range of services of high quality? It was felt that as with most NHS departments, stoma care nursing services could be best served if the stoma care nurse faced up to modern challenges and became involved with decision making processes rather than sitting on the sideline. If nurses took a pro-active role in the developments and drove them, rather than waiting for management or an outside organisation to do so, they would be in a position to influence events and ensure the main aim of producing the best possible and most cost-effective service for their patients (Black 1990).

The first sponsored stoma care nurse was in 1990, in the south of England. When the nurse was told that there was not enough money to continue to finance one of the stoma care posts, she approached one of the ostomy companies for funding. This was the first step in what was to prove a lucrative area for many ostomy companies. At the end of the 1990s, about 60% of stoma care nurses are now sponsored.

In 1991, because of the rise of sponsored posts, not only in stoma care but also beginning to be found in other areas of nursing, wider interest in this phenomenon began to be expressed. The National Audit Office that year produced a report which discussed linked deals and sponsorship of posts. It said that concern had been expressed that these sorts of deals were now becoming commonplace in the NHS. The report objected on three grounds:

- They are usually set up outside supplies control, and are not necessarily subject to full commercial or financial evaluation

- They bypass normal competitive tendering procedures
- They subject NHS staff to pressure from suppliers.

Following the publication of this report more stoma care sponsored posts were established. The next report, *Standards of Business Conduct* (NHSME 1993) was produced. Paragraph 28 of the report stated:

Pharmaceutical companies, for example, may offer to sponsor, wholly or partly, a post for an employing authority. NHS employers should not enter into such arrangements, unless it has been made abundantly clear to the company concerned that the sponsorship will have no effect on purchasing decisions within the authority. Where such a sponsorship is accepted, monitoring arrangements should be established to ensure purchasing decisions are not, in fact, being influenced by the sponsorship agreement.

At the end of 1994 the NHS Executive issued document EL (94)94 which made it clear that the NHS Executive was against any deals with companies until discussions at national level had taken place and the legal situation had been sorted out. In just a few years sponsorship of stoma care nursing posts had come from nowhere to cause many divisive issues among stoma care nurses, ostomy companies and the nurses' managers. Trust managers and finance directors appeared to lose their sense of logic and seemed to believe that there were free nurses and unlimited amounts of cash to be had from ostomy companies. Despite all the national guidelines that had been produced since 1990, Trusts were willing to fly in the face of these guidelines in order to have a so-called 'free' stoma care nurse (Black 1995d). Often the main reason for sponsorship given by a stoma care nurse is that sponsorship is the only way the post and department will survive. For some nurses there is not a choice. If the Trust has gone down this road, because the nurse needs the employment she cannot refuse to be sponsored. In some areas of the UK, stoma care nurses have kept their department in high profile and been proactive and closely followed developments in sponsorship and have worked with their Trusts to keep sponsorship at bay. By educating all areas of the Trust, hospital and community of the perils and pitfalls of commercial sponsorship, these nurses have remained independent and are able to give the patient unrestricted choice of any appliance and service that they may need. From these problems came the Ostomy Patients' Charter (see Appendix), stating the areas of care about which the stoma patient can rightly expect to receive impartial advice.

Quite simply, the main reason for sponsorship of stoma care nurses by interested ostomy companies was that there were clear additional areas where the companies' profits could be enhanced. Although many of the companies entering into sponsorship stated that they were doing it to improve patient care and providing care where there was none, it was the marketing director of one of the companies who told the *Guardian* newspaper, 'if we are making a profit it is logical to stay' (Mihill 1990). What they were saying then was that ostomy companies who sponsor stoma care nurses are seeking a return on their investment.

The sponsorship of stoma care nurses by ostomy companies and NHS managers is mainly funded by the prescription 'on cost' that appliance contractors receive. In effect a retail pharmacist receives a set on cost with an average deduction of 9.67%, effectively making a loss from dispensing appliances. However, the appliance contractor receives up to 25% on cost and this can rise to near 40% if appliances that the manufacturer makes are dispensed and delivered to the patient. In return for this fee the appliance contractor is expected to supply a service and often this is the delivery of the appliances with free material wipes for cleansing the stoma and disposal bags for the used appliance. In some cases there is some nurse support.

In 1993, the Department of Health commissioned Touche Ross to report on the reimbursement and remuneration of appliances. The research was conducted over a period of 2 months, with ostomy companies, appliance contractors, stoma care nurses, patients and patient associations being interviewed (Touche Ross 1994). The report was presented in April 1994 and awaited consideration and implementation. Unfortunately, it seemed to disappear under government changes. In 1998, the NHS Executive took up the subject again and set up an advisory board to look at a review of appliance contractor remuneration and the draft report was begun in December 1998. It was expected among the ostomy industry that the report would appear in the spring of 1999, but due to various reasons, and one in particular – said to be 'the inherent complexities of the issue' – the report will not be available for consultation until the end of 1999 or the Spring of 2000. The expected final outcomes will not now be available until Spring 2001.

At the same time as the current review of appliance contractor remuneration is being carried out, the previous NHS Executive circular *Standards of Business Conduct* (NHSME 1993) is being revised. Ministers have decided that up-to-date guidance should be issued on the NHS ethical standards to be observed when considering commercial sponsorship arrangements. The purpose of the new draft is to emphasise that NHS bodies and primary care staff are accountable for achieving the best possible health care within the resources available, and to advise them to consider fully the implications of a proposed sponsorship deal before entering into any arrangement. The draft advises that local arrangements should be in place so that NHS bodies, members of staff and independent contractors can publicly declare sponsorship and be prepared to be held to account for it.

Patient associations, the nursing profession and health service managers have expressed worries and concerns over ethical issues relating to sponsorship. Stoma care nurses fear that they will have to use less than ideal products because their employer has entered into an exclusive contract with a sponsor. Generally sponsors are attracted to events such as athletics, conferences or financing units or buildings for publicity purposes. They see this as being worthwhile and admirable in its own right. Those who enjoy fruitful working relationships with sponsors would not easily recognise the situations that stoma care nurses in the UK are finding themselves in or find them tolerable.

Black (1995d) suggests that there should be ethical decision making in sponsorship and managers' decisions to accept company money for a nurse should be based on a framework of questions with quantifiable answers:

- As a nurse manager, paragraph 16 of the Code of Professional Conduct should be uppermost in your consideration and you should ensure that neither your nurses' nor your own professional judgement is influenced by any commercial considerations.
- Sponsorship agreements should not take place in a shroud of secrecy in the hope of avoiding criticism or without the consent of the participating nurse.
- Although legislation does not exist specifically stating that a patient's needs must always be put before commercial considerations, the ethical implications involved in the practice of nurse sponsorship may have serious consequences relating to patient care.
- Should you be accepting a long-term relationship with a company, when the company is seeking some sort of exclusive supply agreement or preferential use of its own products?
- Arrangements which appear to give preferential treatment to a company or its products or effectively exclude competitors are likely to infringe UK or European competition law.
- Any initiative which might impair clinical responsibility or inappropriately influence a clinician's choice raises issues of responsibility and accountability for individual patient care.
- Your ethical decision on whether to move to direct sponsorship of stoma care should rest very firmly in the concern that care of this patient group should be determined by need rather than commercial interest.

CONTINUING EDUCATION IN STOMA CARE

It is essential for stoma care nurses today to keep up to date with current nursing practice, both within their specialist area and within nursing in general. Moving into a specialist nursing area does not excuse nurses from keeping up with what is current in general nursing areas. Many nurses, specialist or generic, will throw up their hands in horror at the thought of being 'political', and may consider politics not to be part of nursing. However, what has happened in stoma care with sponsorship shows that it is vital that stoma care nurses know what is happening both inside and outside their speciality. The emphasis by specialist nurses on their difference serves to alienate them from the main body of nursing. Chapman (1983) suggests that it may require a major threat from outside the profession (specialism) to bring about any sense of unity or corporate action.

In 1985 there were two post basic stoma care courses run by the English National Board (ENB) available at several centres in the UK. These were ENB 216, which was aimed at the nurse who expected to move into a post of stoma care nurse, and ENB 980, Principles of Stoma Care, suitable for the ward nurse or the community nurse who wanted to have more knowledge of stoma care but wanted to stay in her role of generic nurse. In 1985 it was felt that specialist nurse education needed to be extended in the light of forthcoming nurse educational changes and the greater responsibility and changing role within the specialism.

In 1996 *Guidelines for the Management of Colorectal Cancer* (Royal College of Surgeons 1996) was published with preparation for surgery stating that the patient who may require a stoma should be seen by a stoma nurse prior to surgery. This was not a new idea to stoma care nurses, but another specialism was seen to be up and coming, that of the colorectal nurse. This nurse was either working in tandem with the stoma care nurse in the same department or in some places as a separate entity. Some were beginning to take an interest in scoping the colorectal patients and following them through their treatment, but patients with stomas would often be passed back to the stoma care nurse. Now for a group of people who were admitted to hospital with colorectal cancer and who would not require a stoma but might need adjuvant therapy, there was a nurse who would be following through their care, just as the stoma care nurse did for stoma patients.

In 1997 the NHS Executive produced clinical outcomes guidelines (COG) on improving outcomes in colorectal cancer (NHS Executive 1997). This was produced in two parts: the research evidence and the manual. The first part provides a summary of systematic reviews of the research evidence relevant to the recommendations made in the manual. The manual recommends that the nursing input for the multidisciplinary team caring for the patient with colorectal cancer is made up of a stoma care nurse, colorectal nurse and palliative care nurse. Although studies were found to identify the value of the palliative care nurse and the stoma care nurse to patients' continuing care, there are no studies or research yet to report on the value of the colorectal nurse to the ongoing care of the patient undergoing colorectal surgery.

There are currently many more ENB courses that can be undertaken by the nurse interested in working towards a diploma or degree with a colorectal pathway (see Box 25.1). They are situated in a limited number of venues around the UK – to find the nearest course contact the ENB.

Box 25.1 Courses available at degree and diploma level

Diploma level
ENB 980 Principles of Stoma Care (30 credits)
R36 Inflammatory Bowel Disease Nursing (30 credits)
ENB 216 Stoma Care Nursing Module 1 (30 credits)

Degree level
ENB 216 Stoma Care Nursing Module 2 (30 credits)
Colorectal Nursing (30 credits)
Inflammatory Bowel Disease Nursing (specialist practice) (30 credits)
Coloproctology Nursing (specialist practice) (30 credits)
Bowel Continence Nursing (specialist practice) (30 credits)
ENB 906 Nursing for Gastrointestinal Endoscopy Assistants (30 credits)

---

that everyone was happy with the situation. Edith had been in hospital now for 2 weeks and was asymptomatic. Edith went down to X-ray but refused to get out of the wheelchair and said she was not having a barium enema. She was returned to the ward.

At the main surgical team meeting Edith was discussed and the consultant said that he was not prepared to undertake surgery on a patient who did not want it. Edith's brother was contacted and told Edith was going back to the home. He was very upset at the fact she was not going to surgery and contacted the consultant again. Until this stage, although everyone had been having discussions about Edith, no meeting had included the stoma therapists who would have substantial input to Edith's care in the hospital and in the community.

Edith's brother was asked by the consultant to contact the stoma therapists to talk about any care Edith would need when surgery was done, and suggested that the stoma therapists contact the home to see how they felt about caring for Edith with a stoma. The home manager was extremely nervous about having Edith back with a stoma and none of the carers had seen one before. The home was promised support and teaching so that everyone would understand about Edith's care and could feel confident with her.

Edith's brother was asked who had signed Edith's consent to surgery and he said that he had. He was asked if he had power of attorney for Edith's affairs or if anyone else in the family did. It appeared that none of the family had power of attorney but just acted in Edith's best interests. The home did not have any legal standing for Edith's affairs and relied on the family.

The senior registrar was keen to operate on Edith the next day but the stoma therapists were not happy with the legal implications and the seriousness of the situation that the hospital could find itself in if the operation went ahead. Because the majority of bowel surgery is done on patients who are not restricted under the Mental Health Act, the question of consent is not a problem. Likewise, because the hospital is a general hospital, patients are not held under any of the statutory powers of the Mental Health Act and therefore the circumstances and safeguards of providing treatment for patients in this group are not commonly used. On consulting with patient affairs they were unsure of the implications for the hospital. It was suggested that the solicitors acting for the hospital were contacted and advice sought.

The solicitors concurred and stated that only the patient could sign consent and power of attorney had no relevance. If the patient's mental condition was felt to be a problem then a doctor who was not involved in the patient's care should assess Edith as to her competence to give consent to any procedure or operation. If the doctor found Edith incompetent to give consent, an application could be made to the court for consent to surgery. If, as it seemed, Edith was refusing to consent to anything, was she therefore incompetent? Ultimately it was decided to discharge Edith back to her home and her carers and either admit her, if necessary, as an emergency and undertake surgery in the first 24 hours, or admit her at a later date and work her up for surgery. At this time an outside opinion would be sought as to her competence to give consent and the mental health team in whose care she had been for several years would also be involved.

EDUCATION

All nurses are aware of the need to keep their post registration requirements up to standard through post registration education and practice (PREP). PREP is about developing individuals in order to maintain and continually improve the standard of care for the patient.

The health care arena is a constantly changing one where nurses have to continually develop their skills and PREP is about keeping up to date in the specialist area that the nurse is working in. There is a basic requirement of 5 days or at least 35 hours of study activity for professional development every 3 years to renew and maintain registration. It is up to nurses to choose the most appropriate study for their personal professional development and it is their responsibility to keep themselves up to date.

There are five broad areas which show a range of activities that can be undertaken by the nurse

and the nurse should ensure that the chosen area meets the needs in the context of practice. These areas are:

1. Patient, client, colleague support (supervision of clinical practice, counselling and leadership in professional practice)
2. Care enhancement (standard setting or new techniques and approaches to care)
3. Practice development (personal research/study or relevant visits to other practice settings)
4. Reducing risk (health promotion or screening)
5. Education development (personal research/study or exchange arrangements).

Stoma care nurses have been in the privileged position of being able to attend frequent study days appropriate to their speciality put on by the ostomy companies. The ostomy companies have made nurse education part of their remit since they see the advantages of having stoma care nurses who are up to date with innovative new surgery, new products, the latest educational initiatives and political changes in nursing. Apart from enabling stoma care nurses to work towards their PREP requirements, stoma care nurses who are up to date are able to offer patients a better standard of care.

Some of the educational modules produced by ostomy companies are intended to assist the stoma therapist to function more effectively in the changes in health care taking place across Europe. The modules are recognised by various universities and awarded points at different levels towards a bachelors or masters degree.

EVIDENCE BASED CARE

The idea of evidence based care (EBC) is not new and people such as Professor David Sackett and his colleagues are stressing that EBC should permeate every clinician's way of thought. The ability to peruse the literature thoroughly and regularly to be able to read and reflect becomes more precious when we all lead such busy and demanding work lives. Knowing how to read and make the best use of medical and nursing literature becomes ever more important. Professor Sackett (Sackett & Haynes 1995) describes evidence based care as: 'the conscientious, explicit and judicious use of current best evidence in making decisions about the care of individual patients.'

It has been suggested that the aim of nursing research and evidence based care is to promote good nursing care and understand the failures of practice with the aim of rectifying the situation. Patients, who are by definition vulnerable and in a relationship with health care professionals in which there is an inherent imbalance of power in favour of the professional, trust nurses to provide the best possible nursing care based on up-to-date knowledge and research. Nurses and health care professionals have no right to intervene in the lives of those in their care, unless they have good reason to think that their interventions will be helpful. Nurses therefore have an obligation to keep their knowledge base and practice skills

up to date by keeping abreast of the literature in their field. This is achieved by reading the literature critically and making balanced judgements about the quality and relevance of the work to their practice (Black 1999a).

RECORD KEEPING

There is a fundamental importance in keeping records as a foundation of care and accurate and up-to-date records present a vital component of high quality care. Poor record keeping undermines patient care and makes the nurse vulnerable to legal and professional problems. Good record keeping promotes the best quality patient care and empowers the nurse to practice to the highest possible standard.

Changes in the NHS give patients greater involvement in making choices about their care, makes the service more patient centred, allows patients access to their records, increases the use of computerised records and enables initiatives such as clinical audit and contracting for health care in the internal market. Today there is increasing litigation within the NHS, with health authorities having to find larger and larger sums of money to pay compensation. When money is paid out in these arenas it can only lead to less money being spent on patient care. In the last decade, the number of professional and legal cases which arose out of poor record keeping escalated dramatically. Records can be required in a court of law months and years after they were written, and good, well-written records will help a hospital in litigious circumstances. Children's and maternity records are kept for 25 years, general nursing records are kept for 8 years. In 1991, 31 practitioners who appeared before the UKCC were struck off for poor record keeping (NHSME 1996).

Many stoma care nurses nowadays use computers to keep patient records. Many of these computers are combined with a sponsored stoma care post and paid for by the sponsoring company. When records are kept in this way they must always be backed up with the disk kept in a safe, fireproof, locked place. Sometimes the software programmes need to be updated by the ostomy company and they will ask to collect the computer and take it away to update. This gesture appears on the face of it to be laudable, but the nurse must be aware that patients' details are on the computer and therefore accessible to the company. A stoma care patient database is extremely valuable to a company as it views the database as new captured data to which mail shots can be sent to try and convert the patient to their appliances. Any upgrading of computer software or hardware should take place in the stoma care department with the stoma care nurse present.

When a new stoma patient is sited and counselled preoperatively, the handwritten notes or computerised notes should state that the siting was with consent of the patient and should also say whether or not written information was given. The medical notes should have the same information recorded in them. The time has come for nurses to be more diligent and organised in their written and verbal communications, and they should always remember the saying 'If it is not recorded it has not been done'.

27

Research and stoma care

Research in stoma care is primarily undertaken to evolve new products for patients, but in the last few years more stoma care nurses are undertaking research projects because they have found an area within their job that they feel could improve patient outcome. Since different perspectives and disciplinary contributions are required, nurse researchers have a vital contribution to make in the evaluation of nursing practice and across the spectrum of health service research. Nurses can, and do, ask questions which are different from those asked by researchers in the biomedical area, and it is this variety of perspectives which brings the very essence of 'difference' to the research. Research does not have to be coterminous with professional or academic boundaries and the theoretical and research methodology should be appropriate to the topic and sufficiently broad to challenge received wisdom and capture data in a variety of ways.

In 1997, the results of a multinational empirical investigation into the view of stoma care nurses about science and research was published (Bullinger et al 1997). It was suggested that stoma care nurses not only needed practical skills in dealing with their patients, but also needed to know about the scientific basis of daily practice. Although the education of stoma care nurses and their working practice differs across Europe, and the degree of importance placed on research by them varies, nonetheless, stoma care nurses are routinely confronted with science in terms of the results of clinical research, or are expected to take part in studies of their own into the evaluation of patient care.

It is estimated that there are about 1673 stoma care nurses working in Europe. Bullinger and colleagues distributed questionnaires to 1100 stoma care nurses at a European conference and received 357 replies. The UK yielded 47 replies and the sociodemographic information showed that the longest time in post was 26 years and the shortest 1 year. The age range was from 30 to 57 years. A total of 21 questions were used to assess experience and interest in science and research.

The overall outcome was useful in understanding the current level of knowledge and information that stoma care nurses have in research and identified areas of expertise. The particular areas of interest identified by stoma care nurses in the questionnaire were:

- Theoretical overviews about the philosophical basis of scientific reasoning
- An overview of research aims and study design
- Practical guidelines on how to conduct research
- Discussion about the relationship between scientific competence and professional status.

Many stoma care nurses will come into contact with and be involved in research trials on new products, not yet on the market, which need to be tested on a human population before being submitted to the drug tariff for general use. Another area which stoma care nurses may be involved in is the evaluation of products which are already on the drug tariff but have only just been released by the company.

TRIALS

In a trial of a new product, an appliance manufacturer will approach several stoma care nurses who have the right population of stoma patients to become part of a multicentre trial to try a new product on specific patients. This might be, for example, patients who have an ileostomy, colostomy or urostomy. The medical department of the ostomy company will have a coordinator who will visit the stoma care nurse to explain the trial and see if there is a suitable population to make the trial viable.

Any clinical trial, whether for a stoma product (usually a new appliance) or for anything else, will need to be approved by an ethics committee, either in a hospital or in the community. The purpose of such an ethical review is to ensure that the interests of the patients who will take part in the study are protected, that the study will have value in terms of benefiting the treatment of other patients, and that the risk/benefit ratio of the study is acceptable.

One aspect of the review of a proposed trial which causes problems for ethics committees relates to informed patient consent. The key words are 'informed' and 'consent'. The prime concern for obtaining informed consent of patients who participate in a trial is to ensure that the patients are fully aware of the nature of the trial, the procedures that will be involved and the potential risks associated with it. Patients must be aware that their participation in the trial is voluntary and that they have the right to refuse to participate without prejudicing their normal medical care. They must be aware that they can withdraw from a trial at any time after it has started without giving a reason why and again that their future care will not be prejudiced.

Patients who participate in a trial must be assured that their privacy will be safeguarded and the data acquired about them will be maintained as confidential information. Information contained in patient records should always be held in confidence and viewed only by those who are directly involved in the patient's care. If the patient records are to be used for research purposes, the prior consent of the patient must be obtained. The relationship of confidence that exists between a clinician and a patient cannot be overturned by a third party, even in the form of a properly constituted ethical committee (RCN 1991b).

When reviewing a consent document, an ethical committee pays particular attention to its wording to ensure that the company has taken into account the intellect of the patients who will be invited to participate. Patients expect any treatment to benefit them and those who participate in clinical trials can rightly expect to derive some benefit. In the context of stoma care with devices and techniques the use of placebos need not arise as far as trials are concerned, but when two devices or techniques are compared, both are expected to provide benefit.

Patient consent is signed with a witness and the patient is also given a patient information sheet with a contact point in case there are any further questions or there is a problem while the trial is being undertaken. The most common problems of consent forms relate to inadequate information about the trial. Ethical committees will reject worthwhile trials because the information is not complete or risks being unintelligible to the patient. Ethical committees need to be assured that patients are able to give informed consent, so that those who read the results of the trial will know that the answer to the question, 'Did the patient give consent?' is 'Yes'.

EVALUATIONS

When a product has been newly launched onto the stoma care market, the sales representative often asks stoma care nurses if they will undertake some evaluations of the appliance on patients in the appropriate group. This is not a trial, since the product is freely available on the drug tariff, but it is a way for the company to introduce the appliance to a wider range of consumers. The number of stoma patients is fairly static and the number of companies wanting their product used becomes ever larger. Evaluations are usually associated with a tick form asking basic questions about the performance of the product. The patient is asked to fill this in and return it to the stoma care nurse when the designated number of appliances have been used. The patient may opt to stay on the product after an evaluation, which is what the company would hope, but some return to the product they were using before the evaluation.

Often, for the evaluation, the stoma care department is offered a fee that can go into the stoma care Trust fund to enable the nurse to have some funding for patient open days, or for the nurse to use towards her professional development. Some Trusts expect stoma care nurses to also raise a sum each year as income generation to help towards the hospital debt. The fee often goes towards conferences or towards the yearly Stoma Care Forum conference. Other uses of evaluation fees are for educational books for the department, slides or other educational aids.

28

The way forward

THE RCN FORUM

The Stoma Care Forum at the Royal College of Nursing was constituted in 1977 as a forum for those working specifically in stoma care and those who have an interest in stoma care. In April 1999 the Stoma Care Forum joined with the RCN Crohn's and Colitis Nursing Special Interest Group, the Endoscopy Associates Group and the Nurse Endoscopist Support and Information Group to become the new RCN Gastroenterology and Stoma Care Nursing Forum. It is being led by new and old members of these groups and the forum will provide an authoritative voice for nurses working in this expanding area of care. As with other forums, it will seek to form relationships with medical and surgical colleagues and to work with them to ensure that patients receive safe and effective care from competent practitioners. The newly formed forum met for its first conference in November 1999 and will give an opportunity for members to network, share ideas, develop policies and improve practice.

THE WORLD COUNCIL OF ENTEROSTOMAL THERAPISTS (WCET)

The World Council of Enterostomal Therapists (WCET), an association of nurses, is an organisation dedicated to the provision of an internationally based corporate identity for qualified enterostomal therapy nurses, the ongoing education of these nurses, and the extension of education related to the needs of individuals with ostomies, incontinence, draining wounds, fistulas, and actual or potential alterations in tissue integrity (WCET 1998).

The WCET provides opportunities for members to meet to discuss matters of common interest related to enterostomal nursing and promotes activities which will assist members to increase their knowledge of, and enhance their contribution to, the subject of enterostomal therapy. There is a conference held worldwide every 2 years and a quarterly journal is produced.

STOMA CARE 2000

In the 1970s, the *Lancet* and the American *Journal of the Medical Association of Georgia* noted in their editorials the rise of the stoma therapist and the new role of the clinical nurse specialist. They felt that the medical and nursing professions generally welcomed the move. Devlin (1980) suggested that this was an attractive role for many nurses wishing to change direction in their clinical career and it was something that the medical profession should encourage. Although there were not many ostomists in the population, their problems at that time were considerable. Perhaps we should take as tongue in cheek his comment that 'surgeons are busy doing other things and operating, and do not have the time to sit and talk to patients or to advise them about the myriad of appliances and services that are now available to them. This is a role that the stoma care nurse can readily fill.'

Today that role has moved on and developed into a group of specialist nurses with skills in business planning, budgeting, research, teaching and excellent patient care for a group of patients who can find themselves on the margins of society because of their changed body status.

Research will have an ever increasing role in stoma care, and although many nurses still see research as being done only by people in ivory towers, the nature and impact of research on stoma therapy will have effects on patient stay, welfare and utilisation of resources. Research draws inferences and important research in stoma care

has to be done by stoma therapists, since people who do not have close contact with ostomists invariably make false assumptions or errors in their research. If research is not shared it is not worthwhile. Many stoma care nurses will have been introduced to research as part of a modular system for a first degree and have a good basis on which to build. There is so much in the clinical practice of stoma care that will provide good research basis, it is surprising that so little is published. The often stated reason that research cannot be undertaken is that stoma care nurses are too busy with their clinical practice and patient case load. However, quality patient care is based on research.

More and more stoma care nurses are called on to justify their position, and over the years the ostomy manufacturers have supported educational initiatives to help stoma care nurses defend their position. Wilson-Barnett (1995) has stressed the lack of experimental evaluations which incorporate an analysis of cost-effectiveness of the specialist nurse, but the Montreux quality of life study is being quoted by GPs as an example of the effectiveness of the stoma care nurse upon the stoma population. However, there is still a general lack of evidence of the effectiveness of specialist nurses at local levels that will demonstrate the research base of their practice.

With the new Gastroenterology and Stoma Care Nursing Forum (see above) there is the potential for dynamic working and research situations among stoma care nurses and their new colleagues and a new source of networking, and at the end of the day this can only be of benefit to the patient.

Since the emergence of the stoma care nurse, doctors, nurses and patients have all reaped benefits from input to this group of patients. As stoma care moves into 2000, stoma care nurses must be ready to evaluate and criticise their own performance by producing research based evidence that will not only strengthen the position of the stoma care nurse but also bring excellence of care to that most important group, stoma patients.

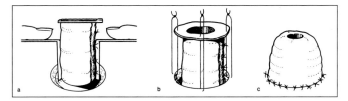

Plate 1 Ileostomy construction

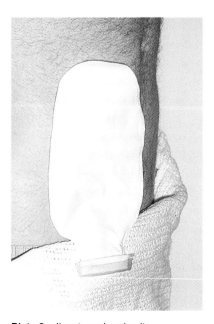

Plate 2 Ileostomy bag in situ

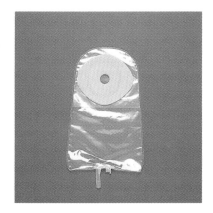

Plate 3 One-piece urostomy bag

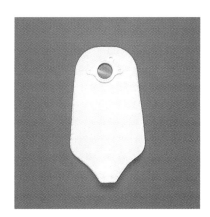

Plate 4 Two-piece urostomy bag

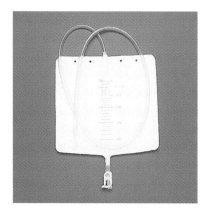

Plate 5 Night drainage bag

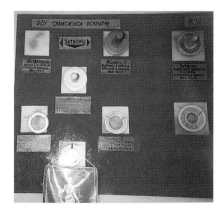

Plate 6 Russian stoma plugs

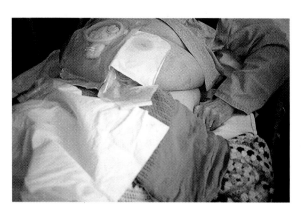

Plate 7 Fistula care

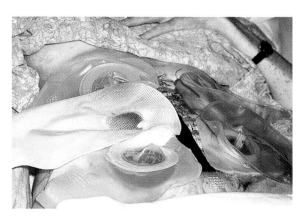

Plate 8 Fistula care

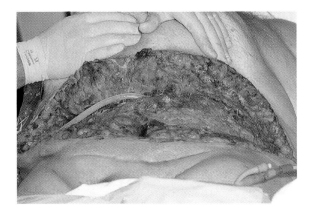

Plate 9 Large wound

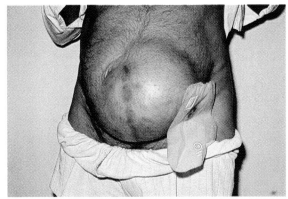

Plate 10 Peristomal hernia

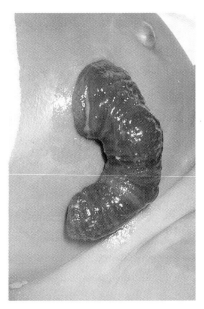

Plate 11 Prolapse

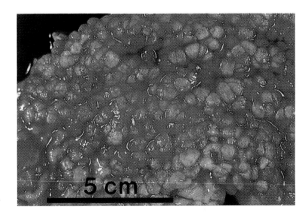

Plate 12 Familial polyposis

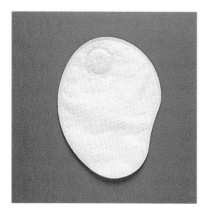

Plate 13 Modern colostomy bag

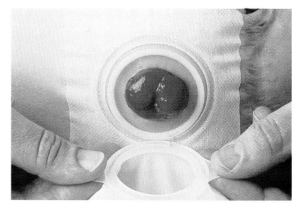

Plate 14 Colostomy and two-piece appliance

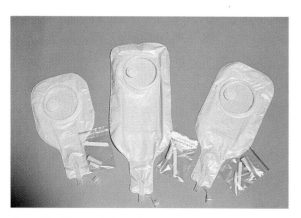

Plate 15 Wound drainage bags

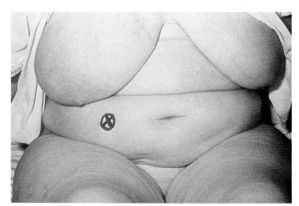

Plate 16 Stoma siting

Appendix

Useful addresses

British Colostomy Association
BCA Office, 13 Station Road, Reading, Berkshire RG1 1LG
Tel: 01743-391537

Ileostomy and Internal Pouch Support Group
PO Box 132, Scunthorpe, DN15 9YW
Tel: 01724-720150

Urostomy Association
Central Office, Beaumont Park, Danbury, Essex CM3 4DE
Tel: 01245-224294

National Association for Colitis and Crohn's Disease
4 Beaumont House, Sutton Road, St Albans,
Hertfordshire AL1 5HH
Tel: 01727-844296

RADAR
12 City Forum, 250 City Road, London EC1V 8AF
Tel: 0207-250-3222

British Digestive Foundation
3 St Andrew's Place, London NW1 4LB

Crohn's in Childhood Research Association
356 West Barnes Lane, Motspur Park, Surrey KT3 6NB

Coeliac Society
PO Box 220, High Wycombe, Buckinghamshire HP11 2HY

NASPCS
National Organiser, 51 Anderson Drive, Valley View Park,
Darvel, Ayr KA17 0DE
Tel: 01560-22024

Cancer Information Service, BACUP
3 Bath Place, Rivington Street, London EC2A 3JR
Tel: 0800-181199

Benefits Agency, Department of Social Security
Tel: 0800-882200

Macmillan Cancer Relief
Anchor House, 15–19 Britten Street, London SW3 3TY
Tel: 0207-351-7811

Sexual and Personal Relationships of the Disabled (SPOD)
286 Camden Road, London N10 3DF
Tel: 0207-607-8851

International Ostomy Association (IOA)
15 Station Road, Reading, Berkshire RG11 1LG

World Council of Enterostomal Therapists (WCET)
c/o Jean Preston, Ashington Hospital, West View,
Ashington, Northumberland NE63 0SA

Royal College of Nursing (RCN)
20 Cavendish Square, London W1M 0AB

Continence Foundation
2 Doughty Street, London WC1N 2PH
Tel: 0207-404-6876

Radiotherapy Action Group Exposure (RAGE National)
24 Lockett Gardens, Trinity, Salford, Manchester M3 6BJ

Ostomy company freephone numbers

AlphaMed	0800 515317
Amcare	0800 885050
Braun Biotrol	0800 163007
Brunlea	0800 834712
Bullens	0800 269327
Coloplast	0800 220622
Convatec	0800 282254
Clinimed	0800 585125
Dansac	0800 581117
Extension 11	0800 521740
Farnhurst Medical	0800 833876
Fittleworth Medical	0800 378846
Hollister	0800 521377
Homecare	0800 243103
Marlen	0800 317602
Novacare	0800 212258
Pelican	0800 318282
Respond Plus	0800 220300
Salt Medilink	0800 626388
SIMS Portex	0800 525350
Thackraycare	0800 590916
UCI Healthcare	0800 7314376
Welland	0800 136213
Wilkinson	0800 626524

Muslim patients and stoma surgery
The effect of religious duties and rituals

Ramadan (fasting)
Physical
Gives increased stamina, but can cause slimming fatigue
Psychological
Self-discipline, will power
Relevance to stoma
Ileostomy: watery, overreacting, dehydration
Colostomy: overeating during sehri, constipation

Namaz (prayer five times per day)
Physical
Al-Wadhu of self, physical exercise
Psychological
Self-audit
Relevance to stoma
Reliable appliance, good skin condition, consider two-piece
appliance

Haj (travel to Mecca)
Physical
Problems of travel, hot weather, tropical diseases
Psychological
Sense of achievement, may be necessary to do after diagnosis
Relevance to stoma
Ileostomy: watery output, dehydration
Colostomy: food change, food poisoning, searching of body
and luggage for drugs
Deterioration of pouches
Contaminated irrigation fluid

OLGA SEARCH FINDINGS

_____ Dimensions of Health _____

QoL Instrument	Coping	Social Integration	Social Contact	Intimacy	Affective Wellbeing	Physical Function
Bowel Disease Q		★		★		★
Coping Inventory (CI)	★					
Social Wellbeing Q (SWBQ)		★				
COOP Chart System (COOP)			★		★	
DUKE-UNC HealthProfile 10 (DUHP10)			★		★	
DUKE-UNC HealthProfile 63 (DUHP63)			★		★	
DUKE HealthProfile (DUKE)			★		★	
Euroqol			★		★	
Functional Status Q (FSQ)			★		★	
Health Utility Index (HUI)			★		★	
Medical Outcome Study (MOS)			★		★	★
MOS Social Support Survey (MOS SSS)			★			
Nottingham Health Profile (NHP)			★		★	★
Quality of Life Package (QLPkg)			★	★	★	
Sched Evain Individ QOL (SEIQOL)			★	★	★	★
Sickness Impact Profile (SIP)			★		★	★
Social Wellbeing Q (SWBQ)			★			
Utility – Category Study (U-CS)			★	★	★	★
Utility – Standard Guide (U-SG)			★	★	★	★
Utility – Time Tradeoff (UTTO)			★	★	★	★
Behaviour Inventory (BI)					★	
Corwell Medical Index (CMI)					★	
Quality Adjusted Life yr. (QALY)					★	★
QoL Q (QLQ)					★	
Symptom Rating Test (SRT)					★	
Disability – Distress Ratio Scale (DDRS)					★	
Quality of Well Being Scale (QWB)					★	★
Quality of Life Index (QLI)			★	★	★	★

FP92A Claim for prescription charge exemption certificate

MEDICAL EXEMPTION

If you suffer from certain medical conditions you are entitled to free NHS prescriptions. But _you need an exemption certificate form FP92_ from your Health Authority to say that you do not have to pay. Use this form to apply to your Health Authority for your exemption certificate.

Use PART 1 to tell your Health Authority about your medical condition, fill in PART 2 overleaf and sign and date the declaration in the spaces provided. Then ask your doctor or the hospital doctor (or your Service Medical Officer if you are a dependant of a member of the Armed Forces) to complete PART 3 overleaf. Your doctor will then send the form to your Health Authority (previously FHSA).

PART 1: ABOUT YOUR MEDICAL CONDITION

I declare that I suffer from: _(tick the box that applies)_,
- ✓ permanent fistula (for example caecostomy, colostomy, laryngostomy or ileostomy) requiring continuous surgical dressing or requiring an appliance
- ✓ epilepsy for which I need continuous anti-convulsive therapy
- ✓ diabetes mellitus except when treated by diet alone
- ✓ myxoedema or other conditions which require supplemental thyroid hormone
- ✓ hypoparathyroidism
- ✓ diabetes insipidus or other forms of hypopituitarism
- ✓ forms of hypoadrenalism (including Addison's disease)

for which specific substitution therapy is essential
- ✓ myasthenia gravis
- ✓ a continuing physical disability which means I cannot go out without the help of another person – temporary disabilities do not count even if they last for several months.

OSTOMY PATIENTS' CHARTER

The ostomy patients' charter presents the special needs of this particular group of people and the care they require.
The stoma patient shall:
- Receive pre-operative counselling to ensure that the patient is fully aware of the risks and benefits of the operation.
- Have a well-constructed stoma placed at an appropriate site, having regard to the comfort of the patient.
- Receive experienced stoma nursing care in the post-operative period.
- Receive full and impartial information about all relevant supplies and products available through the NHS.
- Have the opportunity to choose from a variety of products without prejudice.
- Receive experienced stoma nursing and medical support in both the hospital and community.
- Be given information about the three National Stoma Associations and the advice, counselling and support they can provide.
- Receive support through information to family, carers and friends to increase understanding of the condition and the ability to adjust to the stoma.

WCET HELPFUL HINTS LEAFLETS
HELPFUL HINTS: UROSTOMY

1. Your urostomy is NOT sterile! Wash the stoma and surrounding skin with soap and water, then dry – just as you do the rest of your body

2. You can bath or shower with your pouch (bag) ON or OFF. Dry the skin carefully prior to re-applying your pouch.

3. Avoid the use of bath oils or creams, as this may interfere with the adhesion of the pouch.

4. You may notice a little blood on rubbing the stoma whilst cleaning – this is NORMAL.

5. Keep hairs around the stoma trimmed or shaved. Hold toilet paper over the stoma whilst shaving to protect it.

6. Drink PLENTY of fluids daily – i.e. 6–8 glasses of fluid such as water or tea will keep the urine clear and free from bacterial growth.

7. Some foods may be noted to give the urine an odour – such as asparagus, garlic, fish and onions. This does not mean you cannot enjoy them!

8. Mucous shreds in the urine are NORMAL. Increase your fluid intake if it is severe, and ensure that the mucous does not block the outlet.

9. The best time to change your pouch is in the morning prior to having fluid intake, or after being some three hours without fluid.

10. In hot weather, a cotton pouch cover will help prevent sweating and development of a heat rash under the plastic pouch material.

11. EMPTY your pouch when it is approximately one-third full.

12. Wear pouch INSIDE underwear for added support.

13. Learn the NAME, DIAMETER and type of pouch and skin protection you are wearing – it makes ordering much easier.

14. Always keep a minimum of two weeks' supply in hand – in case of delays.

15. Know where your nearest stomatherapy nurse is based.

16. Ask your stomatherapy nurse for a TRAVELLING OSTOMY CARD with details of your case and stoma supplies when travelling away from home.

17. When travelling, keep your ostomy supplies in your HAND LUGGAGE – not in the aircraft or ship's hold, in case it gets lost. Take a flannel-backed waterproof saver to have between the sheet and the mattress in case of accidents.

18. Watch your weight – any excessive gain or loss can alter the fit and adhesion of your ostomy pouch.

N.B. DON'T BE AFRAID TO ASK QUESTIONS! YOU ARE A SPECIAL INDIVIDUAL – AND ANSWERS PERTAINING TO YOUR RETURN TO WORK, SPORT AND SEXUALITY, WILL BE TAILOR-MADE TO YOU AND YOUR SITUATION.

YOUR LOCAL STOMATHERAPY SERVICE:

STOMATHERAPIST(S): _____

ADDRESS: _____

_____

_____ TEL NO: _____

HELPFUL HINTS: ILEOSTOMY

1. Your ileostomy in NOT sterile! Wash the stoma and surrounding skin with soap and water, then dry – just as you do the rest of your body.

2. You can bath or shower with your pouch (bag) ON or OFF. There is no guarantee that the stoma will not function during this period. Keep some toilet paper handy. Ideally, time this activity when you have NOT just eaten.

3. Avoid the use of bath oils or creams, as they may interfere with the adhesion of the pouch.

4. You may notice a little blood on rubbing the stoma whilst cleaning – this NORMAL.

5. Keep hairs around the stoma trimmed or shaved. Hold toilet paper over the stoma whilst shaving to protect it.

6. Be sure to place SKIN PROTECTION or pouch washer CLOSE to the stoma to avoid getting sore skin from stool contact.

7. Measure your stoma if your skin is getting sore. Perhaps the diameter of your pouch or skin barrier is too large and you will need to cut it SMALLER or, order a smaller diameter ready-sized pouch.

8. 'Wet wipes' or paper tissues make excellent skin cleansers in an emergency.

9. When emptying your pouch, sit 'side saddle', or raise the seat of the toilet, placing some toilet paper in the water to lessen the splash whilst standing or kneeling.

10. Drainable pouches do not require rinsing out, but if you should want to do so, use a syringe or 'Baster' to flush in water via the drainable end.

CAUTION: TOO MUCH WATER LOOSENS THE ADHESIVE AND MAY CAUSE YOU TO LEAK OR SMELL!

11. STRIKE A MATCH before and after releasing gas or stool from your pouch – it is a marvellous (and cheap) deodorant!

12. Always carry a spare pouch with you in case of leaks. Pre-cut everything, and include a disposal bag for the dirty pouch.

13. Keep an extra closure CLAMP in your pocket in case the one you are using breaks (or falls down the toilet!). An elastic band can be used in an emergency.

14. Learn the NAME, DIAMETER and type of pouch and skin protection you are wearing – it makes ordering much easier.

15. Always keep a minimum of two weeks' supply in hand – in case of delays.

16. Know where your nearest stomatherapy nurse is based.

17. Ask your stomatherapy nurse for a TRAVELLING OSTOMY CARD with details of your case and stoma supplies when travelling away from home.

18. When travelling, keep your ostomy supplies in your HAND LUGGAGE – not in the aircraft or ship's hold, in case it gets lost.

19. Watch out for excessive weight gain.

20. Should you get an upset tummy – keep up your fluids and avoid spicy foods and milky products until it settles. You can use 'BLOCKERS' such as IMODIUM, LOMOTIL, CODEINE, KAOLIN. If you do NOT settle within 24 HOURS, CONTACT A DOCTOR or STOMATHERAPY NURSE.

21. ANY CONCERNS OR FEARS YOU MAY HAVE – DON'T HESITATE TO CONSULT YOUR STOMATHERAPY NURSE OR DOCTOR. THEY ARE THERE TO HELP YOU.

N.B. YOU ARE SPECIAL! YOU ARE AN INDIVIDUAL! THEREFORE, QUESTIONS REGARDING RETURNING TO WORK, SPORT AND SEXUAL ACTIVITY, WILL BE INDIVIDUALISED FOR YOUR PARTICULAR CASE. PLEASE ASK FOR ADVICE IF YOU NEED IT.

YOUR LOCAL STOMATHERAPY SERVICE:

STOMATHERAPIST(S): _____

ADDRESS: _____

_____

_____ TEL NO: _____

HELPFUL HINTS: COLOSTOMY
1. Your colostomy is NOT sterile! Wash the stoma and surrounding skin with soap and water, then dry – just as you do the rest of your body.
2. You can bath or shower with your pouch (bag) ON or OFF. There is no guarantee that your stoma will not function, but once a pattern is established, you will find a satisfactory time of day or evening when it will be safest to bath with the pouch off.
3. Avoid the use of bath oils or creams as they may interfere with the adhesion of the pouch.
4. You may notice a little blood on rubbing the stoma whilst cleaning – this is NORMAL.
5. Keep hairs around the stoma trimmed or shaved. Hold toilet paper over the stoma whilst shaving to protect it.
6. There are THREE main types of pouching you will be shown –
   (i) ONE-PIECE CLOSED POUCH
      * ideal for a firm stool.
      * requires changing once or twice daily.
   (ii) TWO-PIECE BASE AND POUCH SET
      * the base may remain on the skin for several days.
      * the pouch can be removed as often as required without damaging the skin.
   (iii) DRAINABLE POUCH
      * ideal for LOOSER stools.
      * allows emptying via clamp at the bottom of the pouch.
      * can remain in place for several days before it needs changing.

YOUR STOMATHERAPIST WILL SHOW YOU – AND WILL RECOMMEND THE BEST FOR YOU.

7. CLOSED-END pouches are best changed when they are half full. Remove the pouch, place in a DISPOSAL BAG, seal and discard in a DUSTBIN. DO NOT FLUSH IT DOWN A TOILET, it may cause a blockage!

8. STRIKE A MATCH before and after releasing gas or stool from your pouch, it is a marvellous (and cheap) deodorant!
9. Drainable pouches do not require rinsing out, but if you should want to do so, use a syringe or 'Baster' to flush in water via the drainable end.

CAUTION: TOO MUCH WATER LOOSENS THE ADHESIVE AND MAY CAUSE YOU TO LEAK OR SMELL!

10. GAS formation can be decreased by AVOIDING gas-producing foods (beans, peas, onions, cabbage) … and chewing the food well. DO NOT cut these foods out of your diet – eat everything – and discuss suitable pouching with your stomatherapy nurse. AIR SWALLOWERS and people who do not 'BURP' very often will pass more GAS INTO THEIR POUCH. Pouches with gas filters are recommended.
11. EAT WELL-BALANCED meals to create a regular bowel pattern.
12. Have an emergency kit with you at all times. Include a spare regular pouch, disposal bag, 'wet wipes' or tissues. When going away, cater for a possible tummy upset and take along some DRAINABLE POUCHES and spare clips, and include a recommended 'BLOCKER' such as IMODIUM, LOMOTIL, CODEINE, KAOLIN.
13. Learn the NAME, DIAMETER and type of pouch and skin protection you are wearing – it makes ordering much easier.
14. Always keep a minimum of two weeks' supply in hand – in case of delays.
15. Know where your nearest stomatherapy nurse is based.
16. Ask your stomatherapy nurse for a TRAVELLING OSTOMY CARD with details of your case and stoma supplies when travelling away from home.
17. When travelling, keep your ostomy supplies in your HAND LUGGAGE – not in the aircraft or ship's hold, in case it gets lost.

N.B. DON'T BE AFRAID TO ASK QUESTIONS! YOU ARE A SPECIAL INDIVIDUAL – AND ANSWERS PERTAINING TO YOUR RETURN TO WORK, SPORT AND SEXUALITY, WILL BE TAILOR-MADE TO YOU AND YOUR SITUATION.

YOUR LOCAL STOMATHERAPY SERVICE:

STOMATHERAPIST(S): _____

ADDRESS: _____

_____

_____ TEL NO: _____

References

Allen R, Steinberg D M, Alexander Williams J, Cooke W T 1977 Crohn's disease involving the colon: an audit of clinical management. Gastroenterology 73: 723–732

Allingham H 1891 Inguinal colotomy. British Medical Journal ii: 337–338

Allison M 1995 Comparing methods of stoma formation. Nursing Standard 9(24): 25–28

Allison M 1996 Discharge planning for the person with a stoma. In: Myers C (ed) Stoma care nursing. Arnold, London

Amyand 1735 Cited in Lichtman A L, McDonald J R 1944 Fecal fistula. Surgical Gynaecology and Obstetrics 78: 449–468

Bekkers M, van Knippenberg F, van den Borne H, Poen H, Bergsma J, van Berge Hengouwen G 1995 Psychosocial adaptation to stoma surgery. Journal of Behavioural Medicine 18(1): 1–31Bell 1972

Bergstrand O, Hellers G 1983 Breast feeding during infancy in patients who later develop Crohn's disease. Scand J Gastroenterol 18: 903–906

Berwick D 1989 Continuous quality improvements in health care. Journal of Nursing Quality Assurance

Black P 1987 The appliance of science. Community Outlook, May

Black P 1988 The role of the stoma care nurse. Unpublished paper given to the Ministry of Health, Prague, Czechoslovakia

Black P 1989a An introduction to stoma care. Clinical Pharmacology Research Institute, Folkestone

Black P 1989b Complications associated with a stoma. Surgical Nurse 2(6): 1–4

Black P 1989c Family adaptation and the care of the stoma patient. Primary Health Care 7(7): 4–5

Black P 1989d Pre and post operative care of the stoma patient. Unpublished paper given to the Institute of Proctology, Moscow, USSR

Black P 1990 Stoma care in the community. Nursing Standard 4(43): 54–55

Black P 1992 Body image after enterostomal surgery. Unpublished MSc Thesis, Steinberg Collection, Royal College of Nursing, London

Black P 1994a Choosing the correct appliance. British Journal of Nursing 3(11): 545–550

Black P 1994b History and evolution of stomas. British Journal of Nursing 3(1): 6–11

Black P 1994c Hidden problems of stoma care. British Journal of Nursing 3(14): 707–711

Black P 1994d RCN Nursing Update. Learning Unit 045. Nursing Standard 8(34): 3–13

Black P 1994e The role of the stoma care nurse. Pharmacy Update. Chemist and Druggist, 21 May

Black P 1995a Sponsorship in stoma care. BSTA Bulletin No. 20

Black P 1995b Sponsorship in stoma care. British Journal of Health Care Management 1(13)

Black P 1995c Stoma care after hospital discharge. Nurse Prescriber/Community Nurse, July

Black P 1995d Stoma care: finding the most appropriate appliance. British Journal of Nursing 4(4): 188–192

Black P 1995e The body politic. Paper given to the third European Congress of Stoma and Continence Care, Rotterdam, Holland

Black P 1995f Caring for large wounds and fistulas. Journal of Wound Care 4(1): 23–26

Black P 1995g Pharmacists and stoma care nurses form a caring partnership. Pharmacy in the Community. The NPA Review

Black P 1996a Stoma skin care. Practice Nursing 7(10): 32–34

Black P 1996b Stoma appliances: what's new? Nurse Prescriber/Community Nurse, April

Black P 1996c Choice cuts. Nursing Times 8(92): 28–30

Black P 1997a Familial adenomatous polyposis. Eurostoma 18: 8–9

Black P 1997b Life carries on: stoma aftercare. Practice Nursing 8(4): 29–34

Black P 1997c Practical stoma care: a community approach. British Journal of Community Health Nursing 2(5): 249–253

Black P 1998a Audit is central to modern nursing. Eurostoma, 24 September

Black P 1998b Overcoming stoma problems. Nurse Prescriber/ Community Nurse, September

Black P 1999a Evidence based healthcare. Fifth European Congress for Nurses with an Interest in Stoma Care, 11–14 May 1999, Copenhagen, Denmark

Black P 1999b In: Heywood Jones I UKCC Code of Professional Conduct: a guide for nurses. Scutari Press, Harrow, Middlesex

Boarini A 1989 Principles of stoma care for infants. Journal of Enterostomal Therapy 16(1): 21

Bonarparte B 1979 Ego depressiveness, open mindedness, and nurse attitudes toward culturally different patients. Nurs. Res. 28: 166–172

Borwell B 1997 Developing sexual helping skills. Medical Projects International, Berkshire

Boykoe E, Perera D, Koepsell T et al 1988 Effects of cigarette smoking on the clinical course of ulcerative colitis. Scandinavian Journal of Gastroenterology 23: 1147–1152

Breckman B 1981 Stoma care. Beaconsfield Publishers, Beaconsfield, Buckinghamshire

Bricker E 1950 Bladder substitution after pelvic evisceration. Surg. Gynaecol, and Obstet. 30: 1511–1512

Brooke B 1952 The management of ileostomy including its complications. Lancet ii: 102–104

Bullinger M, Tille S, Dumrese C, Ptjens S 1997 Science and research: the view of stoma care nurses. European Research Journal: A Supplement to Eurostoma, March, Issue 1

Bulow S, Holm N, Hague M 1986 The incidence and prevalence of familial polyposis coli in Denmark. Scand J Soc Med 14: 67–74

Butler C 1952 Some observations on the treatment of carcinoma of the rectum. Proceeding

Busutill-Leaver R 1992 So you've heard about it, but what is a Mitrofanoff? Talkabout: 12. Simcare, West Sussex

Busutill-Leaver R 1994a The Mitrofanoff pouch: a continent urinary diversion. Professional Nurse August: 748–753

Busutill–Leaver R 1994b Cranberry juice. Professional Nurse 11: 525–526

Butler C 1952 Some observations on the treatment of carcinoma of the rectum. Proceedings of the Royal Society of Medicine 45: 41–50

Calnan J 1988 Towards a conceptual framework of lay evaluation of health care. Social Science and Medicine 27: 927–933

Cancer Research Campaign 1993 Cancer of the large bowel. Fact Sheet 18.1. Cancer Research Campaign, Information Unit, Coulsize Terrace, London NWI 4JL, UK

Capra F 1982 The turning point: science, society and the rising culture. Collins, London

Castledine G 1982 Just like Topsy the job grew. Nursing Mirror 155: 48

Chapman C 1983 Unity with diversity within the nursing profession. Journal of Advanced Nursing 8: 245–247

Chapman R, Foran R, Dunphy J 1964 Management of intestinal fistulas. Am J Surg 108: 157–164

Cheselden W 1784 Anatomy. London

Cohen F, Lazarus R 1982 Coping with the stresses of illness. In: Stone G C (ed) Health psychology. Jossey-Bass, London

Colo News 1997 Where next with rectal cancer? 6(1) May

Coloplast 1995 Ostomy and ostomy patients: an introductory guide. Coloplast, Peterborough, Cambridgeshire

CORCE 1997 Stoma siting. Medical Projects International, Maidenhead, Berkshire

CoTui F 1930 Kaolin in the treatment of external gastro-intestinal fistulas. Ann Surg 91: 123–125

Cousins N 1989 Head first: the biology of hope. Penguin, New York

Cripps N 1993 Incidence and screening for early diagnosis. Proceedings from 'Changing Habits': a review of bowel cancer. Macmillan, Basingstoke

De Ridder D 1997 Nutritional guidelines for stoma patients. Eurostoma 18: 14–15

Department of Health 1993 Improving clinical effectiveness. EL(93). Department of Health, London

Department of Health and Social Services 1978 The provision of stoma care. HMSO, London

Devlin H B, Plant J A, Griffin M 1971 Aftermath of surgery for anorectal cancer. British Medical Journal iii: 413–418

Devlin B 1980 Stoma therapy review. Coloplast, Peterborough

Devlin B 1985 Second opinion. Health and Social Services Journal 1: 82

Devlin B, Plant J 1979 Sexual function: an aspect of stoma care. British Journal of Sexual Medicine 6: 33–37

Dinnick T 1934 The origins and evolution of colostomy. British Journal of Surgery 22: 142–154

Dixon C F, Deuterman J L 1938 The management of external intestinal fistulas. Journal of the American Medical Association 111: 2095–2101

Dixon C, Benson R 1946 Principles in the management of external fecal fistulas. Journal of the American Medical Association 130: 755–761

Douglas M 1966 Purity and danger: an analysis of the concepts of pollution and taboo. Penguin, Harmondsworth

Douglas M 1975 Implicit meanings. Routledge and Kegan Paul, London

Dowd C N 1917 Enterostomy for ileus. Annals of Surgery: 45: 95–194

Druss R 1969 Psychological response to colectomy. Archives of General Psychiatry 20: 419–427

Dudley H 1978 If I had carcinoma of the middle third of the rectum. British Medical Journal 1: 1035–1067

Dudrick S J, Wilmore D W, Vars H M, Rhoads J E 1968 Long term total parenteral nutrition with growth, development and positive nitrogen balance. Surgery 64: 132–134

Dukes C 1947 Management of a permanent colostomy. Lancet iii: 12–14

Dunkel-Schetter C 1984 Social support and cancer: the findings based on patient interviews and their implications. Journal of Social Issues 40(4): 77–98

Dunlop M 1986 Is a science of caring possible? Journal of Advanced Nursing 11: 661–670

Edmunds L, Williams G, Welch C 1960 External fistulas arising from the gastrointestinal tract. Annals of Surgery 152: 445–471

Eisenberg L 1977 Disease and illness: distinctions between professional and popular ideas of sickness. Culture, Medicine and Psychiatry 1: 9–23

Eliason M 1993 Cultural diversity in nursing care: the lesbian, gay or bisexual person. Journal of Transcultural Nursing 5(1): 14–20

Farbrother M 1993 What can I eat? Nursing Times 89: 14, 63

Festinger L 1964 The motivating effect of cognitive dissonance. In: Harper R, Christansen C, Hunka S The cognitive processes: readings. Prentice Hall, Englewood Cliffs, New Jersey, pp 509–523

Fillingham S, Douglas J 1997 Urological nursing. Baillière Tindall, London

Finlay I, McArdle 1986 Occult hepatic metastases in colorectal carcinoma. British Journal of Surgery 73: 732–735

Fleming J 1984 Bags of choice. Senior Nurse 1(23): 1009

Foucault M 1976 The birth of the clinic. Tavistock, London

Franceschi S, Panza E, La-Vecchia C et al 1987 Non specific inflammatory bowel disease and smoking. Am J Epidemiol 125: 445–452

Frazer J G (1922) 1994 The golden bough. Chancellor Press, London (first published 1922, Macmillan, London)

Gerhardt U 1989 Ideas about illness: an intellectual and political history of medical sociology. Macmillan Education, Hampshire

Gilat T, Langman M, Rozen P et al 1986 The genetics and epidemiology of inflammatory bowel disease. Karger, Basel

Gill T, Feinstein A 1994 A critical appraisal of the quality of life measurements. Journal of the American Medical Association 272: 619–626

Girard M 1988 Technical expertise as an ethical form: towards an ethics of distance. Journal of Medical Ethics 14: 25–30

Goffman E 1963 Stigma. Pelican, London

Goffman E 1969 The presentation of self in everyday life. Allen Lane, London

Goldsmith H 1961 Control of viscerocutaneous fistulas by a new suction device. New England Journal of Medicine 23: 1052–1054

Goldsmith H S 1967 The management of viscerocutaneous fistulas. Surgery 61: 361–363

Goligher J C 1971 Resection with extericrisation in the management of faecal fistulas originating in the small intestine. British Journal of Surgery 58: 163–167

Good B 1981 The heart of what's the matter: the semantics of illness in Iran. Culture, Medicine and Psychiatry 1: 25–58

Gowers S 1981 Clinical nurse specialists: something special. Nursing Mirror 152: 30–33

Guyatt G, Cook D 1994 Health status, quality of life, and the individual patient. Journal of the American Medical Association 272: 630–631

Guyot M, Samardizic M, Heinrichs E et al 1992 Stomahesive in peristomal skin care. Bristol-Myers Squibb Group, Paris

Hallisey M 1995 Palliative chemotherapy in gastric and colorectal cancer. Journal of Cancer Care 4: 131–133

Hampton B, Bryant R 1992 Ostomies and continent diversions: nursing management. Mosby Year Book, St Louis

Hamric A, Spross J 1983. The clinical nurse specialist in theory and practice. Grune and Stratton, Orlando, Florida

Hannestead V 1995 The management of entero-cutaneous fistulas by ETs. Eurostoma, Spring

Harries A, Jones L, Heatley R et al 1982 Smoking habits and inflammatory bowel disease. British Medical Journal 284: 1161

Hartmann H 1923 Congrès Français de Chirurgie 30: 411

Heister L 1743 A general system of surgery in 3 Parts. Part 1, p 63, part 2, p 53

Hellers G, Bergstrand D, Ewerth S, Holstrom B 1980 Occurrence and outcome after primary treatment of anal fistulae in Crohn's disease. Gut 21: 525–527

Helman C 1990 Culture, health and illness. Wright, London

HMSO 1974 Disposal of household wastes. HMSO, London

Holmes S 1996 Making sense of cancer chemotherapy. Nursing Times 92(36): 42–43

Horhammer 1916 Cited in Rinsema W 1992 Gastrointestinal fistulas. Datawyse, Maastricht

Jefferies E 1993 At home with stoma care. Nursing Times 89(14): 59–62

Johnson H 1992 Stoma care for infants, children and young people. Paediatric Nursing, May: 8–11

Jones D, Irving M 1993 ABC of colorectal diseases. BMJ Publishing Group, UK

Jones Heywood I 1999 UKCC Code of Conduct: a critical guide. EMAP Nursing Times, London

Kagan C, Evans J 1995 Professional interpersonal skills for nurses. Chapman and Hall, London

Kelly M 1985 Loss and grief reactions as responses to surgery. Journal of Advanced Nursing 10: 517–525

Kelly M 1991 Coping with an ileostomy. Social Science and Medicine 33: 115–125

Kelly M 1992 Colitis. Routledge, London

Kelly M, Henry T 1992 A thirst for practical knowledge. Professional Nurse 7(6): 350–351, 354–356

Kleinman A 1980 Patients and healers in the context of culture: an exploration on the borderland between anthropology, medicine and psychiatry. University of California Press, Berkeley, California

Klopp A 1990 Body image and self concept among individuals with stomas. Journal of Enterostomal Therapy 17(3): 98–105

Kmietowicz Z 1997 Are you prepared for the measles vaccine debate? Nurse Prescriber/Community Nurse, August: 31–34

Knowles G, Jodrell D 1997 Recent developments in adjuvant chemotherapy for colorectal cancer. European Journal of Cancer Care 6: 18–22

Kocher H M, Saunders M P 1999 Complacency or ignorance about rectal bleeding. Colorectal Disease 1(6): 332–333

Kock N 1969 Intra-abdominal reservoir in patients with permanent ileostomy. Archives of Surgery 99: 223–231

Krumm S 1982 Psychological adaptation of the adult with cancer. Nursing Clinics of North America 17: 729–737

Lahey F 1951 Indications for surgical intervention in ulcerative colitis. Annals of Surgery 133: 726–742

Landrum B 1998 Marketing innovations to nurses. Part 2: Marketing's role in the adoption of innovations. Wound, Ostomy and Continence Nursing 25(5): 227–232

Laney M L 1969 Hope as a healer. Nursing Outlook 17: 45–46

Langman M 1990 Epidemiology of inflammatory bowel disease. Hospital Update March: 243–246

Larrey D 1823 Some observations on wounds of the intestines: surgical essays. Trans. Revere J Maxwell, Baltimore

Leaper D, Cameron S, Lancaster J 1987 Antiseptic solutions. Community Outlook April 14: 30–34

Leaver R 1993 What is a Mitrofanoff? Talkabout (Simcare Publications) 12: 10

Lederman J 1997 Funding issues in the treatment of cancer. Royal College of Physicians, London

Lee M 1985 The future role of stoma care nursing. A report of a seminar held in Copenhagen, Medical Education Services Ltd

Lenninger M 1978 Transcultural nursing: concepts, theories and practices. Wiley, New York

Lenninger M 1985 Qualitative research methods in nursing. Grune & Stratton Inc., London

Leslie C 1976 Asian medical systems: a comparative study. University of California Press, Berkeley, California

Levi-Strauss C 1963 Structural anthropology. Basic Books, New York

Lewis D, Pewick R 1933 Faecal fistula. Int Clin 43: 111–130

Lewis G 1981 Cultural influences on illness behaviour. In: Eisenberg L, Kleinman A (eds) The relevance of social science for medicine. Reidel, Dordrecht

Lichtman A, McDonald J 1944 Fecal fistula. Surg Gynecol Obstet 78: 449–468

Littlewood J 1985 No flag day for incontinence. Self Health September: 32–34

Littlewood J 1989 A model of nursing using anthropological literature. International Journal of Nursing Studies 23: 221–229

Littlewood J, Holden P (eds) 1991 Anthropology and nursing. Routledge, London

Littré M 1732 Histoire de l'Académie Royale des Sciences. Paris, pp 36–37

Livingstone J 1997 Personal communication. Mount Vernon Hospital

Loudon J 1977 The anthropology of the body. Academic Press, New York

Lynch H, Lanspa S, Bowman B et al 1988 Hereditary non-polyposis colorectal cancer: Lynch syndromes I and II. Gastroenterology Clinics of North America 17: 679–712

McConnell R, Rozen P, Langman M J S, Gilat T (eds) 1986 The genetics and epidemiology of inflammatory bowel disease. Basel: Kager

MacDonald L D, Anderson H R, Bennett A E 1984 Stigma in patients with rectal cancer: a community study. Journal of Epidemiology and Community Health 38: 284–290

McKee L 1996 Sponsored stoma care doubles the cost to the GP. Pulse 28 September

McSharry M 1995 The evolving role of the clinical nurse specialist. British Journal of Nursing 4(11): 641–646

McWhinney I R, Bass M J, Donner A 1994 An evaluation of a palliative care service: problems and pitfalls. British Medical Journal 309: 1340–1342

Majeed A 1998 Using Pact to audit prescribing of stoma care products. Clinical Care, General Medicine. National Association of Fundholding Practices Yearbook

Markham G 1988 Special cases: a broad look at the development of clinical nurse specialists. Nursing Times 84(26): 29–30

Marks R, Evans E, Clarke T 1978 The effects on normal skin of adhesives from stoma appliances. Current Medical Research and Opinion 5(9): 720–725

Massey A 1997 New innovative treatment in metastatic colorectal cancer. International Journal of Palliative Nursing 3(3): 171–174

Maule W 1994 Screening for colorectal cancer by nurse endoscopists. New England Journal of Medicine 330: 183–187

Mayo C, Schlicke C 1941 The surgical management of faecal fistulae. Annals of Surgery 114: 1011–1017

Mead J 1994 An emphasis on practical management. Professional Nurse 9(6): 405–410

Melville A, Sheldon T, Gray R, Snowden A 1998 Management of colorectal cancer. Journal of Quality in Health Care 7: 103–108

Mihill C 1990 Gift wrapped nursing under fire. Guardian 18 May

Miller L 1995 The clinical nurse specialist: a way forward. Journal of Advanced Nursing 22: 494–501

Mitrofanoff P, Bonnet O, Annoot N et al 1992 Continent urinary diversion using an artificial sphincter. British Journal of Urology 70: 26–29

Montreux Study 1998 Quality of life study in stoma patients. ConvaTec Europe, Ickenham, Middlesex

Motley R S, Rhodes L, Ford G A 1987 Time relationships between cessation of smoking and onset of ulcerative colitis. Digestion 37: 125–127

Motley R, Rhodes J, Williams G et al 1990 Smoking eicosanoids and ulcerative colitis. Journal of Pharmacy and Pharmocology 42: 288–289

MRC/UKCCR 1997 Colorectal cancer trials. Colonews 6(1): 1–4

Murray R 1972 Principles of nursing intervention for the adult patient with body image changes. Nursing Clinics of North America 7(4): 697

Nasmyth D 1984 Comparison of defunctioning stomas: a prospective controlled trial. British Journal of Surgery 71(11): 909

National Audit Office 1991 National Health Service supplies in England. Report by the comptroller auditor general. HMSO, London

Nemhauser G, Brayton D 1967 Enterocutaneous fistulas involving the jejuno-ileum. Am Surg 33: 16–20

NHS Executive 1994 Executive letter 94/94. DOH, Leeds

NHS Executive 1997 Improving outcomes in colorectal cancer: the research evidence. DOH, London

NHS Executive 1999 Commercial sponsorship: ethical standards for the NHS. HSC 1999/999. NHS Executive, Leeds

NHSME 1993 Standards of business conduct for NHS staff. January, para 28

NHSME 1996 Keeping the record straight. NHS Training Directorate

Nicholls R J, Loboski O Z 1987 Restorative proctocolectomy: the four loop (W) reservoir. British Journal of Surgery 74: 564–566

Noddings N 1984 Caring: a feminine approach to ethics and moral education. University of California Press, Berkeley, California

Nordstrum H, Hulten L 1987 Loop ileostomy as an alternative to transverse loop colostomy. Journal of Enterostomal Therapy 10(3): 92–94

Notter J 1995 Marketing specialist practice to managers and purchasers. British Journal of Nursing 4(22): 1330–1334

Oberst M, Scott D 1988 Post discharge distress in surgically treated cancer patients and their spouses. Research in Nursing and Health 11(23): 223

Ogilvie W 1944 Abdominal wounds in the Western Desert. Surgery, Gynecology and Obstetrics 78: 225–238

Orbach C, Tallent N 1965 Modification of perceived body and body concepts. Archives of General Psychiatry 12: 126–135

Orem D 1991 Nursing concepts of practice. Mosby Year Book, St Louis

Osborne M, Stansby G 1994 Smoking and chronic inflammatory bowel disease. Journal of the Royal Society of Health 317–319

Ostomy Patients' Charter (see Appendix)

Padilla G, Grant M 1985 Quality of life as a cancer nursing outcome variable. Advances in Nursing Science 8: 45–60

Parent W 1995 In: Hunt G (ed.) Ethical issues in nursing. Routledge, London, p 43

Parkes C 1972 Bereavement: studies of grief in adult life. Pelican, Harmondsworth

Parks A G, Nicholls R J 1978 Proctocolectomy without ileostomy for ulcerative colitis. British Medical Journal ii: 85–88

Parks A, Nicholls R, Belliveau P 1980 Proctocolectomy with ileal reservoir and anal anastomosis. British Journal of Surgery 67: 533–538

Patey D 1951 Primary epitheleal apposition in colostomy. Proceedings of the Royal Society of Medicine 44: 423–444

Patey D, Fergusen J, Exley M 1946 Gravity drainage in the prone position in the treatment of digestive fistulae of the abdominal wall. British Medical Journal 30: 814–815

Paul F 1895 Colotomy. Liverpool Medico-Chirugical 15: 374–388

Persson P G, Ahblom A, Hellers G 1990 Inflammatory bowel disease and tobacco smoke: a case control study. GUT 31: 1377–1381

Phillips S 1995 Supporting the patient with inflammatory bowel disease. Nursing Times 91(27): 38–39

Plant J A, Devlin B 1975 Disposal of disposable colostomy appliances. British Medical Journal ii: 705

Plumley S 1939 Care of ileostomy: how one patient worked out his own care. American Journal of Nursing 39: 257–259

Potter C A 1929 Treatment of duodenal and faecal fistula. Further observations. Journal of the American Medical Association 92: 359–363

Price B 1990 Body image: nursing concepts and care. Prentice Hall, Hertfordshire

Pringle W, Swan E, Wade B 1997 Continuing care for stoma patients. Paper given to the RCN Stoma Care Forum

Pullan R 1994 Colonic mucus, smoking and ulcerative colitis. Surgical England 78: 85–91

Qureshi B 1988 Transcultural medicine. Kluwer Academic Publishers, London

Rampton D, McNeil N, Sarner M 1983 Analgesic ingestion and other factors preceding relapse in ulcerative colitis. Gut 24: 187–189

Randles J 1992 An alternative to urinary conduit. Nursing Standard 6(46): 33–36

RCN 1988 Specialities in nursing. RCN, London

RCN 1990 Congress resolution RCN Stoma Care Forum Newsletter 10: 2

RCN 1991a Nursing, the nature and scope of professional practice. Issues in Nursing and Health, No. 1. RCN, London

RCN 1991b Patients records and research: a position statement. Issues in Nursing, No. 2. RCN, London

RCN 1994 Guidelines on commercial sponsorship of nursing posts. Issues in Nursing, No. 9. RCN, London

Reissman F 1965 The 'helper' therapy principle. Social Work 10: 27–32

Righter B 1995 Uncertainty and the role of credible authority during ostomy experience. Journal of Wound, Ostomy and Continence Nursing 23(2): 100–104

Rinsema W 1992 Gastro-intestinal fistulas. Datawyse, Maastricht, The Netherlands

Robertson-Smith W 1889 Lectures on the religion of the Semites, 3rd edn. Macmillan, New York

Roe B 1993 Catheter associated urinary tract infections: a review. Journal of Clinical Nursing 2: 97–203

Royal College of Surgeons of England and the Association of Coloproctology of Great Britain and Ireland 1996 Guidelines for the management of colorectal cancer.

Rubin P, Devlin B 1987 The quality of life with a stoma. British Journal of Hospital Medicine 38(4): 300–306

Rutegard J, Dahlgren S 1987 Transverse colostomy or loop ileostomy as diverting stoma in colorectal surgery. Acta Chir Scand 153: 229–232

Sackett D L, Haynes B 1995 On the need for evidence based medicine. Evidence Based Medicine 1: 4–5

Samuelson S M 1976 Ulceros colit och prokit. Thesis, University of Uppsala, p 128

Scott G 1990 In: Hunt G Ethical issues in nursing. Routledge, London, p 43

Slevin M 1996 Adjuvant treatment for colorectal cancer. British Medical Journal 13: 392–393

Smaje C 1995 Health, race and ethnicity: making sense of the evidence. King's Fund Institute, London

Sobota A 1984 Inhibition of bacterial adherence by cranberry juice: a potential use for the treatment of urinary tract infections. Journal of Urology 131: 1013–1016

Sontag S 1978 Illness as metaphor. Vintage, New York

Spector R 1977 Health and illness among ethnic people of colour. Nurse Educator May–June: 10–13

Spigeleman A, Thompson J 1994 Introduction, history and registries. In: Phillips R, Spiegleman A, Thompson J (eds) Familial adenomatous polyposis and other polyposis syndromes. Edward Arnold, London

Stafford Miller 1993 Ulcerative colitis: about your condition. Stafford Miller, Welwyn Garden City, Hertfordshire

Strauss A, Strauss S 1944 Surgical treatment of ulcerative colitis. Surgical Clinics of North America 24: 211–244

Stringer M 1985 Patient population and appliance technology trends. The Future Role of Stoma Care Nursing, Copenhagen. Medical Education Services Ltd

Stuchfield B, Boyles A, Eccersley A, Williams N S 1997 The gracilis neosphincter operation. Royal London Hospital, Issue 6

Sutherland A, Orbach C, Dyk R et al 1952 Psychological impact of cancer and cancer surgery: adaptation to colostomy. Cancer 5: 857–872

Taylor I Robertson A 1994 The health needs of gay men: a discussion of the literature and implications for nursing. Journal of Advanced Nursing 20(3): 560–566

Tenopyr J, Shafiroff B 1937 High intestinal fistula: method of treatment. Annals of Surgery 105: 477–480

Todd I 1978 Sexual relationships and childbirth. In: Intestinal stoma. Heinemann Medical, London

Tomey A M, Alligood M R 1998 Nursing theorists and their work. Mosby Year Books, St Louis

Touche Ross 1994 Reimbursement and remuneration of appliances. DOH, London

Trainor M 1981 Acceptance of ostomy and the visitor role in a self-help group for ostomy patients. Nursing Research 31(2): 102–106

Turnburg L 1989 Clinical gastroenterology. Blackwell Scientific, Oxford

Turnbull R, Turnbull G 1991 The history and current status of paramedical support for the ostomy patient. Seminars in Colon and Rectal Surgery 2(2): 131–140

Turner V 1967 The forest of symbols. Cornell University Press, Ithaca

Tysk C, Jarnerot G 1992 Has smoking changed the epidemiology of ulcerative colitis. Scand J Gastroenterol 27: 508–512

UKCC 1992 Code of Professional Conduct. UKCC, London

UKCC 1994 The future of professional practice: standards for education and practice following registration. UKCC, London

UKCC 1996 Guidelines for professional practice. UKCC, London

UKCC 1997 PREP and you. UKCC, London

Van Gennep A 1909 Les reites de passage. Paris. (Translated London 1960)

Vessey M, Jewell D, Smith A et al 1986 Chronic inflammatory bowel disease, cigarette smoking and use of oral contraceptives: findings of a large cohort study of women of child bearing age. British Medical Journal 292: 1101–1103

Von Miculicz 1903 Chirurghische erfahrungen uber das Darmcarcinom. Archiv fur Klinische Chirurgie 69: 28–47

WCET 1998 Members' handbook. World Council of Enterostomal Therapists, Central Office, Ontario

Wade B 1989 A stoma is for life. Scutari Press, Harrow

Wade B 1990 Colostomy patients: psychological adjustment at 10 weeks, 1 year after surgery in districts which employed stoma care nurses and districts which did not. Journal of Advanced Nursing 15: 1297–1304

Wade B, Moyer A 1989 An evaluation of clinical nurse specialists: implications for education and the organisation of care. Senior Nurse 9(9): 11–15

Wallace D 1970 Uretero-ileostomy. British Journal of Urology 42: 529–534

Webster P 1985 Special babies. Community Outlook July 1984: 19–22

Williams N, Johnston O 1983 The quality of life after rectal excision for low rectal cancer. British Journal of Surgery 70: 460–462

Wilson E, Desrisseaux B 1983 Stoma care and patient teaching. In: Wilson-Barnett J (ed) Recent advances in nursing. Vol 6: Patient Teaching. Churchill Livingstone, Edinburgh

Wilson J 1996 A tool for minimising risk. Multidisciplinary Pathways of Care series. Health Care Risk Report, March

Wilson-Barnett J 1995 Specialism in nursing: effectiveness and maximization of benefit. Journal of Advanced Nursing 21: 1–2

Wilson-Barnett J, Beech S 1994 Evaluating the clinical nurse specialist: a review. International Journal of Nursing Studies 31(6)

Young A 1982 The anthropologies of illness and sickness. Ann Rev Anthropol 11: 257–285

Zimmer J G, Groth-Juncker A, McCusker J 1984 Effects of a physician-led home care team on terminal care. Journal of American Geriatric Society 32: 288–292

Zimmer J G, Groth-Juncker A, McCusker J 1985 A randomized controlled study of a home health care team. American Journal of Public Health 75: 134–141

Further reading

Borwell B 1997 Developing sexual helping skills. Medical Projects International, Maidenhead, Berkshire

Fillingham S, Douglas J 1997 Urological nursing. Baillière Tindall

Gerhardt U 1989 Ideas about illness. Macmillan Education, Hampshire

Hampton B G, Bryant R A 1992 Ostomies and continent diversions. Mosby Year Book, St Louis

Helman C 1990 Culture, health and illness. Butterworth

Kelly M 1992 Colitis. Routledge, London

Price B 1990 Body image: nursing concepts and care. Prentice Hall, London

Tomey A M, Alligood M R 1998 Nursing theorists and their work. Mosby Year Book, St Louis

Index